Intrinsic Muscles of the Hand

Guest Editor

STEVEN GREEN, MD

HAND CLINICS

www.hand.theclinics.com

February 2012 • Volume 28 • Number 1

SAUNDERS an imprint of ELSEVIER, Inc.

W.B. SAUNDERS COMPANY
A Division of Elsevier Inc.

1600 John F. Kennedy Blvd. • Suite 1800 • Philadelphia, Pennsylvania 19103

http://www.theclinics.com

HAND CLINICS Volume 28, Number 1
February 2012 ISSN 0749-0712, ISBN-13: 978-1-4557-3869-4

Editor: David Parsons
Developmental Editor: Teia Stone

Hand Clinics (ISSN 0749-0712) is published quarterly by Elsevier Inc., 360 Park Avenue South, New York, NY 10010-1710. Months of publication are February, May, August, and November. Business and Editorial Offices: 1600 John F. Kennedy Blvd., Ste. 1800, Philadelphia, PA 19103-2899. Customer Service Office: 3251 Riverport Lane, Maryland Heights, MO 63043. Periodicals postage paid at New York, NY and at additional mailing offices. Subscription price is $368.00 per year (domestic individuals), $583.00 per year (domestic institutions), $184.00 per year (domestic students/residents), $420.00 per year (Canadian individuals), $666.00 per year (Canadian institutions), $500.00 per year (international individuals), $666.00 per year (international institutions), and $243.00 per year (international and Canadian students/residents). Foreign air speed delivery is included in all *Clinics* subscription prices. All prices are subject to change without notice. **POSTMASTER:** Send address changes to *Hand Clinics*, Elsevier Health Sciences Division, Subscription Customer Service, 3251 Riverport Lane, Maryland Heights, MO 63043. Customer Service (orders, claims, online, change of address): Elsevier Health Sciences Division, Subscription Customer Service, 3251 Riverport Lane, Maryland Heights, MO 63043. Tel: 1-800-654-2452 (U.S. and Canada); 314-447-8871 (outside U.S. and Canada). Fax: 314-447-8029. E-mail: journalscustomerservice-usa@elsevier.com (for print support); journalsonlinesupport-usa@elsevier.com (for online support).

Reprints. For copies of 100 or more of articles in this publication, please contact the Commercial Reprints Department, Elsevier Inc., 360 Park Avenue South, New York, New York 10010-1710. Tel.: 212-633-3812; Fax: 212-462-1935; E-mail: reprints@elsevier.com.

Hand Clinics is covered in *MEDLINE/PubMed (Index Medicus)*, *Current Contents/Clinical Medicine*, *EMBASE/Excerpta Medica*, and *ISI/BIOMED.*

Printed and bound by CPI Group (UK) Ltd, Croydon, CR0 4YY

Transferred to Digital Print 2012

Contributors

GUEST EDITOR

STEVEN GREEN, MD
Associate Clinical Professor of Orthopaedic
Surgery, New York University and Mount
Sinai Schools of Medicine; Associate Chief,
Division of Hand Surgery, NYU-Hospital for
Joint Diseases, New York, New York

AUTHORS

BASIL R. BESH, MD
Surgery of the Hand and Upper Extremity,
Chairman of Orthopedics, Washington
Hospital, Fremont, California

JACK CHOUEKA, MD
Chairman, Department of Orthopedic Surgery,
Maimonides Medical Center, Brooklyn;
Assistant Clinical Professor, Department
of Orthopedic Surgery, New York University
School of Medicine, New York, New York

STEVEN GREEN, MD
Associate Clinical Professor of Orthopaedic
Surgery, New York University and Mount
Sinai Schools of Medicine; Associate Chief,
Division of Hand Surgery, NYU-Hospital for
Joint Diseases, New York, New York

SALIL GUPTA, MD
Clinical Assistant Professor, Department of
Orthopedic Surgery, NYU-Hospital for Joint
Diseases, New York, New York

DEEPAK KAPILA, MD
Plantation, Florida

STEVE K. LEE, MD
Associate Professor of Orthopaedic Surgery,
Hand and Upper Extremity Surgery Service,
Hospital for Special Surgery, Weill Cornell
Medical College, New York, New York

PAM LEVINE, MD
Brooklyn, New York

FREDERIC E. LISS, MD
Malvern, Pennsylvania; Chairman and Director,
Physicians Care Surgical Hospital, Royersford,
Pennsylvania; Phoenixville Orthopedic
Associates, PC, Surgery of the Hand and
Upper Extremity, Phoenixville, Pennsylvania

HEIDI MICHELSEN-JOST, MD
Jackson, Wyoming

NADER PAKSIMA, DO, MPH
Associate Professor of Orthopedic Surgery,
New York University; Assistant Chief of the
Hand Service, New York University; Chief
of Orthopedic Surgery, Jamaica Hospital,
New York University-Hospital for Joint
Diseases, New York, New York

RAM PALTI, MD
Department of Hand Surgery, Sheba Medical
Center, Ramat Gan, Israel

MICHELE PASQUALETTO, OTR/L, CHT
Outpatient Occupational Therapy Department,
Hospital for Joint Diseases, NYU Langone
Medical Center, New York, New York

JOHN A. PASQUELLA, DO
Hand Fellow, Department of Hand Surgery,
New York University-Hospital for Joint
Diseases Institute, New York, New York

MARTIN A. POSNER, MD
Chief, Division of Hand Surgery, New York
University–Hospital for Joint Diseases,
New York, New York

ANTHONY SAPIENZA, MD
Assistant Professor, Orthopaedic Surgery,
Hand Surgery Division, NYU-Hospital for Joint
Diseases; Co-Chief of Hand Surgery Service,
Bellevue Hospital Center, New York, New York

SUSAN CRAIG SCOTT, MD
Assistant Clinical Professor, Department
of Orthopedic Surgery, New York University
School of Medicine, New York, New York

MONICA SEU, OTR/L, CHT
Outpatient Occupational Therapy Department,
Hospital for Joint Diseases, NYU Langone
Medical Center, New York, New York

MORDECHAI VIGLER, MD
Department of Orthopaedic Surgery,
Rabin Medical Center, Hasharon Hospital,
Petach-tikva, Israel

JAMIE R. WISSER, MD, FACS
Clinical Assistant Professor of Orthopaedic
Surgery, Division of Hand Surgery, NYU/
Langone Medical Center, New York, New York;
Princeton Surgical Specialties, PA, East
Windsor, New Jersey

Contents

Preface xi

Steven Green

Anatomy and Function of the Thenar Muscles 1

Salil Gupta and Heidi Michelsen-Jost

> The four thenar muscles make up the intrinsic muscles of the thumb. They include the abductor pollicis, adductor pollicis, opponens pollicis, and flexor pollicis brevis. Thumb motion is facilitated through the coordination of these intrinsic muscles. The thumb musculature dynamically allows for precision pinching ad power gripping.

The Interosseous Muscles: The Foundation of Hand Function 9

Frederic E. Liss

> The interosseous muscles of the hand can be thought of as the cornerstone of hand function, as they provide a "foundation" for all intrinsic and extrinsic hand movements. Innervated by the ulnar nerve and organized in dorsal and palmar layers, these pivotal muscles have small excursion yet great impact on finger balance, grip, and pinch function, particularly when impaired by denervation and/or contracture. This article gives an overview of the functional anatomy and pathologic dysfunction of the interosseous muscles within the context of this *Hand Clinics* issue on the intrinsic muscular function of the hand.

Anatomy and Function of Lumbrical Muscles 13

Ram Palti and Mordechai Vigler

> The lumbrical muscles are unique in having their origin and insertion on tendons. The lumbricals assist in metacarpophalangeal joint flexion; they contribute to interphalangeal joint extension by acting as deflexors of the proximal interphalangeal joint. Anatomically, they are highly specialized in terms of their architectural properties, with a small physiologic cross-sectional area but long fiber length. Their unique properties indicate that they are probably important in fast, alternating movements and fine-tuning digit motion.

Anatomy and Function of the Hypothenar Muscles 19

John A. Pasquella and Pam Levine

> The hypothenar eminence is the thick soft tissue mass located on the ulnar side of the palm. Understanding its location and contents is important for understanding certain aspects of hand function. Variation in motor nerve distribution of the hypothenar muscles makes surgery of the ulnar side of the palm more challenging. To avoid injury to nerve branches, knowledge of these differences is imperative. This article discusses the muscular anatomy and function, vascular anatomy, and nerve anatomy and innervation of the hypothenar muscles.

Restoration of Opposition 27

Martin A. Posner and Deepak Kapila

> Opposition is not grasp but a preposition for grasp that involves 3 components of thumb movements: abduction, flexion, and pronation. Thumb opposition is usually

lost with paralysis of the thenar muscles innervated by the median nerve. Many op-position transfers have been described that differ in the donor tendon, route of trans-fer, and method of attachment to the thumb. No one transfer is applicable for every clinical condition, and each transfer has its advantages and disadvantages. Many factors must be evaluated to decide if surgery is likely to be beneficial and then de-cide on the optimum treatment.

Restoration of Pinch in Intrinsic Muscles of the Hand   45

Steve K. Lee and Jamie R. Wisser

The primary intrinsic muscles responsible for key and tip pinch are the adductor pol-licis, first dorsal interosseous and flexor pollicis brevis muscles. Numerous condi-tions can lead to their dysfunction. Non-operative treatment consists of exercises of the compensating extensor pollicis longus and flexor pollicis longus muscles and use of adaptive devices, such as larger grips. Operative treatments include ten-don transfers and joint fusions. The most common tendon transfer procedures in-clude transferring of the extensor carpi radialis brevis to the adductor pollicis muscle or transfering of the abductor pollicis longus to the first dorsal interosseous muscle. Both require use of extension tendon grafts. In cases of joint instability or arthrosis, arthrodesis of the thumb and index finger MP or IP joints, alone or in com-bination, may be indicated.

Correction of the Claw Hand   53

Anthony Sapienza and Steven Green

Intrinsic paralysis can be the manifestation of a variety of pathologic entities (stroke, cerebral palsy, Charcot-Marie-Tooth, muscular dystrophy, leprosy, trauma, cervical disease, and compressive and metabolic neuropathies). Patients present with a spectrum of clinical findings dependent on the cause and severity of the disease. The 3 main problems caused by intrinsic weakness of the fingers are clawing with loss of synchronistic finger flexion, inability to abduct/adduct the digits, and weak-ness of grip. Clawing is defined as hyperextension of the metacarpophalangeal joints and flexion of the interphalangeal joints. This article describes the clinical eval-uation and surgical treatment options for claw hand.

Intrinsic Contractures of the Thumb   67

Jack Choueka and Susan Craig Scott

A wide range of conditions can lead to intrinsic contractures of the thumb. A thor-ough understanding of the normal and pathologic anatomy as well as the disease processes and their effect on thumb function is essential in understanding and treat-ing these contractures. Because intrinsic contractures of the thumb rarely present in isolation, a patient-specific approach based on functional needs is required. Preven-tion of iatrogenic contractures and progression of predictable contractures regard-less of etiology is the health care provider's primary responsibility.

Intrinsic Contractures of the Hand   81

Nader Paksima and Basil R. Besh

Contractures of the intrinsic muscles of the fingers disrupt the delicate and complex balance of intrinsic and extrinsic muscles, which allows the hand to be so versatile and functional. The loss of muscle function primarily affects the interphalangeal joints but also may affect etacarpophalangeal joints. The resulting clinical picture is often termed, *intrinsic contracture* or *intrinsic-plus hand*. Disruption of the balance between intrinsic and extrinsic muscles has many causes and may be secondary to changes within the intrinsic musculature or the tendon unit. This article reviews diagnosis, etiology, and treatment algorithms in the management of intrinsic contractures of the fingers.

Hand Therapy for Dysfunction of the Intrinsic Muscles

87

Monica Seu and Michele Pasqualetto

Intrinsic muscle dysfunction can be devastating. Patients often have difficulty using the affected hand for most daily activities. Physicians, occupational therapists, and patients have to work together to enable the patient to regain functional use of the hand to perform activities that are a part of their life roles. Occupational therapists play an important role in the rehabilitation process to regain motion, strength, and dexterity so that patients can use the hand more functionally. Patient education and active participation in their therapy is also essential in the functional recovery of the hand.

Index

101

Hand Clinics

FORTHCOMING ISSUES

May 2012

Elite Athlete's Hand and Wrist Injury
Michelle Carlson, MD, *Guest Editor*

August 2012

Emerging Technology in Management of Disorders of the Hand
Jeffrey Yao, MD, *Guest Editor*

November 2012

Arthroplasty Around the Wrist
Marwan A. Wehbé, *Guest Editor*

RECENT ISSUES

November 2011

Hand Transplantation
Gerald Brandacher, MD, and
W.P. Andrew Lee, MD,
Guest Editors

August 2011

New Advances in Wrist and Small Joint Arthroscopy
David J. Slutsky, MD,
Guest Editor

May 2011

Elbow Arthritis
Julie E. Adams, MD, and
Leonid I. Katolik, MD,
Guest Editors

February 2011

Current Concepts in the Treatment of the Rheumatoid Hand, Wrist and Elbow
Kevin C. Chung, MD, MS, *Guest Editor*

THE CLINICS ARE NOW AVAILABLE ONLINE!

Access your subscription at:
www.theclinics.com

Preface

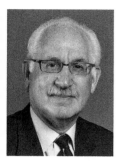

Steven Green, MD
Guest Editor

"There is a general tendency to curtail progressively the time allotted to the teaching of anatomy in the medical schools, but the need for anatomy is greater than ever. It is essential in surgery, where an adequate knowledge of structure could have eliminated inadequate operations performed in the past and those still being performed."

This quote from Emanuel Kaplan, MD in his introduction to his classic book "Functional and Surgical Anatomy of the Hand" is more true today than when first published in 1953. During the more than 30 years of mentoring medical students, residents, and postgraduate hand fellows, I remain impressed with their lack of knowledge and confusion concerning the structure and function of the intrinsic muscles of the hand and the methods of evaluation and treatment of the various disorders that affect these critical muscles. The purpose of this issue of the *Hand Clinics* is to provide a comprehensive review of the intrinsic muscles, their structural and functional anatomy, the effect of their dysfunction, and the various methods that can be used for rehabilitation.

All of the authors of this monograph are members of the Kaplan Hand Club, comprising hand surgeons associated with the NYU-Hospital for Joint Diseases because of either their postgraduate training in the Division of Hand Surgery or their activity on the teaching faculty. This issue is dedicated to three brilliant surgeons who have served as chiefs of Hand Surgery at this hospital. The first is Emanuel Kaplan, who was the first hand surgeon at HJD. He was a dedicated comparative anatomist, teacher, and surgeon. Besides his famous book mentioned above, he also translated another classic: "Physiology of Motion," written by Duchenne in 1866. Richard Smith succeeded Dr Kaplan and was also a superb teacher, surgeon, and author. His publications about the anatomy, function, and disorders of the intrinsic muscles remain unrivaled classics. Sadly his book on tendon transfers is no longer in print. Our present chief is Martin Posner and was my first teacher of Hand Surgery and has been my office mate, great friend, and fishing buddy for more than 30 years. He has been responsible for training 83 fellows and countless residents. Like his predecessors, he is internationally known for his insight, comprehensive knowledge, masterful teaching, and technical skill.

It is my hope that the readers of this issue of the *Hand Clinics* will obtain a greater understanding of the unique and complex function of the intrinsics and will find themselves better prepared to evaluate and treat disabilities caused by disorders of these muscles.

Steven Green, MD
2 East 88th Street
New York, NY 10128, USA

E-mail address:
Stevengreenmd@aol.com

Hand Clin 28 (2012) ix
doi:10.1016/j.hcl.2011.09.007
0749-0712/12/$ – see front matter © 2012 Elsevier Inc. All rights reserved.

Anatomy and Function of the Thenar Muscles

Salil Gupta, MD[a,*], Heidi Michelsen-Jost, MD[b]

KEYWORDS

- Thenar • Pollicis • Adductor pollicis • Opponens • Pollicis
- Abductor pollicis brevis • Flexor pollicis brevis

On the length, strength, free lateral motion, and perfect mobility of the thumb, depends the power of the human hand. Without the fleshy ball of the thumb, the power of the fingers would avail nothing; and accordingly the large ball, formed by the muscles of the thumb, is the distinguishing character of the human hand

—*Charles Bell[1]*

The hand is an important functioning organ requiring rest and performing the greatest part of activities, including locomotion, if need be. The function of the entire upper extremity is to position the hand in space. The arm and forearm position the hand so that we can perform essential tasks. In all its spatial locations, the hand not only grasps and releases various objects but transports them as well. Moreover, through the hand, as through sight and hearing, we form a conception of the outside world. It is truly the extension of our brain into the surrounding world; it is the mirror of our innermost response to the outside world…The most characteristic features of the human hand are the comparative length of the thumb. The longer thumb of humans permits better opposition.

—*Emmnuel B. Kaplan and Morton Spinner[2]*

It is in the motion and function of the thumb that the thenar muscles play their anatomic role. There are four intrinsic muscles of the thumb: abductor pollicis brevis (APB), opponens pollicis (OPP),

flexor pollicis brevis (FPB), and adductor pollicis (ADD). Three of these muscles, APB, OPP, and FPB, form the fleshy mass at the radial border of the palm. Most of the thenar muscles originate partly from the transverse carpal ligament. Their insertions are primarily on the base of the thumb proximal phalanx, except for the opponens, which inserts on the first metacarpal (**Figs. 1–4, Table 1**).

FUNCTIONAL MOVEMENTS OF THE THUMB

To fully appreciate the actions of the thenar muscles, the complex motions of the thumb must be understood. Thumb motion is facilitated through the coordination of intrinsic thenar and extrinsic musculature. The thumb musculature dynamically allows for precision pinching and power gripping. Because thumb stability is actively maintained by muscles rather than by articular constraints, most muscles attached to the thumb tend to be active during most thumb motions.[3]

The opposable thumb is indispensible to man. "The important function of the thumb is its movement in opposition to the index finger, and to the other fingers."[4] A thumb in true opposition is not only opposite the fingers, but it is far forward from them and is rotated, so the pulp faces the fingers and nail parallels the palm.[5] Opposition is a rotational movement of the first metacarpal around the long axis of its shaft. The motion of opposition "consists of rotation of the volar surface of the thumb so that from a normal position of rest, perpendicular to the transverse plane of the hand, it is able to face the volar surface of

---

The authors have nothing to disclose.

[a] Department of Orthopedic Surgery, NYU-Hospital for Joint Diseases, 95 University Place, 8th Floor, New York, NY 10003, USA
[b] PO Box 7434, Jackson, WY 83002, USA
* Corresponding author.
E-mail address: salilnyc@hotmail.com

Hand Clin 28 (2012) 1–7
doi:10.1016/j.hcl.2011.09.006

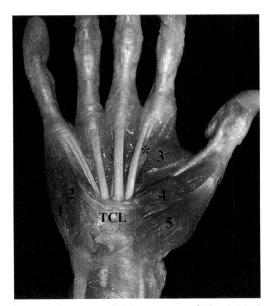

Fig. 1. Palmar superficial exposure of the intrinsic muscles of the hand. The transverse carpal ligament (TCL) serves as an origin for the flexor digiti minimi (2), the FPB (4), and the APB (5). Abductor digiti minimi (1). Lumbrical muscle (*asterisk*). The ADD (3) is seen deep to the thenar musculature, its broad origin along the volar radial margin of the long finger metacarpal. (*From* Leversedge F, Goldfarb C, Boyer M. Hand. In: A pocket manual of hand and upper extremity primus manus. Philadelphia: Wolters Kluwer Lippincott Williams & Wilkins; 2010. p. 28; with permission.)

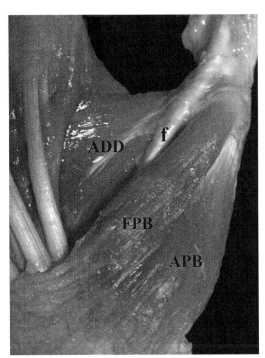

Fig. 2. Palmar view of the thenar musculature. The APB and the FPB muscles originate from the transverse carpal ligament. The FPB origin is more distal than that of the APB. The flexor pollicis longus tendon (f) emerges from the interval between the deeper ADD and the FPB or APB. (*From* Leversedge F, Goldfarb C, Boyer M. Hand. In: A pocket manual of hand and upper extremity primus manus. Philadelphia: Wolters Kluwer Lippincott Williams & Wilkins; 2010. p. 28; with permission.)

the fingers after pulling out completely (abduction) from the surface of the palm. Thus, it produces a rotatory motion from the 90° of rest to 180° parallel with the transverse plane of the hand."[3] Opposition involves the combined motions of flexion, pronation, and palmer abduction of the thumb metacarpal. Reposition, the opposite of opposition, involves, extension, supination, and adduction of the thumb metacarpal.

Abduction is moving the thumb anterior to, or away from, the palm. Adduction is the motion bringing the thumb metacarpal toward the second metacarpal, in the plane of the palm. Flexion is the action of moving the thumb in an ulnar direction within the plane of the palm. The thumb, therefore, can be flexed in full abduction, full adduction, or anywhere in between. Extension is the opposite motion of flexion.

ANATOMY

The most important functional determinant of a muscle is its architecture, the arrangement of muscle fibers relative to the axis of force

generation.[6] Muscle excursion is directly proportional to muscle fiber length. The force generated by a muscle is directly proportional to its cross-sectional area. Several investigators have studied the various physiologic properties of the thenar muscles and a summary of their findings is found in **Tables 2–4**.[6,7]

Despite their small size, the intrinsic muscles are very efficient because of their direct line of pull between origin and insertion.[8] The actions of muscles are determined by their insertions, the course and direction of their tendons, and their relation to the joints and ligaments. To appreciate the function of a muscle, the details of its anatomy must be understood.[9]

The APB

Abductor means "to draw away from." It is derived from the Latin ab, meaning "away from," and ducere, meaning "to draw." The word pollicis for thumb is derived from pollex, thumb (see **Figs. 1–4**, **Table 1**).[10–12] The APB is a subcutaneous muscle

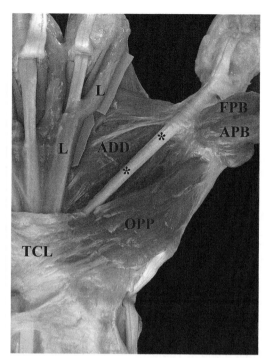

Fig. 3. Palmar view of the deep thenar musculature relationships with reflection of the FPB and APB muscles. The OPP originates from the transverse carpal ligament (TCL), the trapezium, and the thumb carpometacarpal joint capsule and inserts into the volar-radial distal thumb metacarpal. Flexor pollicis longus tendon (*asterisk*). ADD. Lumbrical to the index (L). (*From* Leversedge F, Goldfarb C, Boyer M. Hand. In: A pocket manual of hand and upper extremity primus manus. Philadelphia: Wolters Kluwer Lippincott Williams & Wilkins; 2010. p. 29; with permission.)

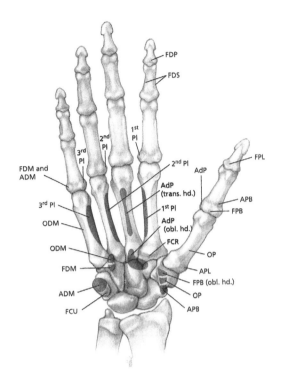

Fig. 4. Origin (*red*) and insertions (*blue*) of thenar muscles. ADM, abductor digiti minimi; AdP, adductor pollicis; AdP (obl. Hd.), adductor pollicis oblique head; AdP (trans. hd.), adductor pollicis transverse head; APB, abductor pollicis brevis; APL, abductor pollicis longus; FCR, flexor carpi radialis; FCU, flexor carpi ulnaris; FDM, flexor digit minimi; FDP, flexor digitorum profundus; FDS, flexor digitorum superficialis; FPB (obl. hd.), flexor pollicis brevis oblique head; FPL, flexor pollicis longus; ODM, opponens digiti minimi; OP, opponens pollicis; PL, palmaris longus. (*From* Botte MJ. Muscle anatomy. In: Doyle JR, Botte MJ, editors. Surgical anatomy of the hand and upper extremity. Philadelphia: Lippincott Williams & Wilkins; 2003. p. 112; with permission.)

on the proximolateral aspect of the thenar eminence.[10,13–16] The APB lies radial to the FPB in the superficial aspect of the thenar eminence. The APB provides the shape and contour of the radial side of the thenar eminence.[10] It arises primarily from the transverse carpal ligament, with some fibers arising from the scaphoid tubercle, trapezium, and the tendon of the abductor pollicis longus.[10,13,17–19] The muscle is divided into two lamellae.[14] By way of a thin flat tendon, its medial, or deep, fibers insert onto the radial base of the thumb proximal phalanx, as well as to the lateral side of the capsule of the metacarpophalangeal joint (MCPJ), and the radial sesamoid.[4,13,17,18] Its fibers blend with those of the adjacent FPB.[13,15,20] The superficial lateral fibers insert into the aponeurosis of the extensor pollicis longus.

The abductor APB is innervated by the recurrent branch of the median nerve (95%) or ulnar nerve (2.5%) or by dual innervation (2%).[17,18,21,22] The median nerve branch enters the deep aspect of the muscle in its middle third and can have several

different branching patterns.[14,23,24] The vascular supply of the APB is from the superficial palmer branch of the radial artery, which arises from the radial artery at the level of the radial styloid, and often by a separate and discreet branch arising directly from the radial artery as it lies on the radial border of the thumb.[13–15]

Anomalies of the APB include the muscle having additional heads, varying attachments to the radial styloid, ADD, OPP, palmaris longus, extensor carpi radialis longus, or flexor pollicis longus.[10,14,16]

The primary function of the APB is the abduction and flexion of the thumb metacarpal, performing the action of pulling the thumb away from the palm at a right angle to the palm of the hand. In addition, the muscle functions to extend the thumb interphalangeal joint, through its extensor pollicis longus insertions, and ulnarly deviates the MCPJ.[10,13,17,18]

Table 1
Summary of thenar muscle anatomy and function

Muscle	Origin	Insertion	Primary Action	Innervation
APB	Trapezium, Scaphoid	Lateral base thumb proximal phalanx, extensor mechanism	Abduction, Opposition	Median nerve. C8-T1
OPP	Trapezium	Anterolateral first metacarpal	Pronation	Median nerve. C8-T1
FPB Superficial Head	Transverse carpal ligament, Trapezium	Lateral base thumb proximal phalanx	Flexion of Metacarpophalangeal joint	Median nerve. C8-T1
FPB Deep head	Second metacarpal	Lateral base thumb proximal phalanx	Flexion of Metacarpophalangeal joint	Ulnar nerve. C8-T1
ADD Oblique Head	Capitate, Second or third metacarpals	Medial base thumb proximal phalanx	Adduction	Ulnar nerve. C8-T1
ADD Transverse Head	Distal half third metacarpal	Medial base thumb proximal phalanx	Adduction	Ulnar nerve. C8-T1

The APB produces abduction and flexion of the metacarpal, slight flexion of the proximal phalanx, and extension of the distal phalanx; pronation of the entire thumb occurring through the CMC joint is simultaneous with flexion of the thumb metacarpal. These actions produce opposition.[9,10,14,16] "The APB alone is able to produce excellent opposition of the thumb, and it is the most important muscle of the thenar group. By virtue of its insertion into the base of the proximal phalanx and into the long extensor, this muscle can stabilize the MCPJ in abduction, flexion, and pronation and can assist extension of the terminal phalanx, -the essential functional components of opposition."[25] This action is enhanced with the help of the OPP.[9]

The OPP

The term *opponens* is Latin for the action of movement against or toward an opposing structure (see Figs. 3 and 4, Table 1).[10–12] The OPP is a short, thick, triangular sheet of muscle that lies beneath the abductor pollicis brevis. It originates from the carpometacarpal joint capsule, the tubercle of the trapezium, and the transverse carpal ligament. It fans out to insert on the volar radial length of the thumb metacarpal. The vascular supply of the muscle is via the superficial palmar branch of the radial artery; branches from the first palmar metacarpal artery, princeps pollicis, and radialis indicis arteries; and the deep palmar arch.[13–15,17–19]

Innervation patterns for the OPP show significant variability. It is innervated by the recurrent branch of the median nerve (83%) or ulnar nerve (9%) or by dual median and ulnar innervation (7.5%).[17,18,21,22,26] Forrest[27] found that the OPP is innervated by the median nerve exclusively in 20 out of 25 hands and that dual innervation with

Table 2
Muscle area and force

Muscle	Mean Muscular Surfaces (cm²)	Standard Deviation	Force (kg)
APB	1.30	.62	13
OPP	1.92	0.85	19.2
FPB	1.18	.54	11.8
ADD	3.73	1.21	37.3

Data from Fahrer M. The thenar eminence: an introduction. In: Tubiana R, editor. The hand. Philadelphia: W.B. Saunders; 1981. p. 257.

Table 3
Muscle contraction and work capacity

Muscle	Mean Range of Contracting (mm)	Standard Deviation	Work Capacity (meters-kilogram)
APB	40.60	10.48	0.52
OPP	21.70	6.52	0.40
FPB	41.90	11.8	0.49
ADD	40.40	5.91	1.5

Data from Fahrer M. The thenar eminence: an introduction. In: Tubiana R, editor. The hand. Philadelphia: W.B. Saunders; 1981. p. 258.

Table 4
Architectural properties measured

Muscle	Muscle Mass (g)	Muscle Length (mm)	Fiber Length (mm)	Cross-Sectional Area (cm^2)	Fiber Length-Muscle Length
APB	2.61 ± 1.19	60.4 ± 6.6	41.6 ± 5.6	0.68 ± 0.28	0.69 ± 0.09
OPP	3.51 ± 0.89	55.5 ± 5.0	35.5 ± 5.1	1.02 ± 0.35	0.64 ± 0.07
FPB	2.58 ± 0.56	57.2 ± 3.7	41.5 ± 5.2	0.66 ± 0.20	0.73 ± 0.08
ADD	6.78 ± 1.84	54.6 ± 8.9	340 ± 7.5	1.94 ± 0.39	0.63 ± 0.15

Data from Jacobson MD, Raab R, Fazeli BM, et al. Architectural design of the human intrinsic hand muscles. J Hand Surg Am 1992;17:806.

the median and ulnar nerves occurs in 5 out of 25 hands. Harness and colleagues[28] found dual innervation in 77% of their patients, whereas 23% had innervation only from the median nerve. Anomalies of the OPP include coalescence with the FPB, extra heads of the muscle, and (rarely) complete absence.[14]

The OPP flexes and pronates the thumb metacarpal.[16–18] The OPP "initiates the movement of opposition at the level of the first metacarpal."[29] The OPP enhances the work of opposition of the APB.[9]

The FPB

The Latin term flexor means "that which bends," derived from flexus, "bent" (see **Figs. 2–4, Table 1**).[10–12] The FPB has two heads, a superficial (lateral), and a deep (medial). The superficial head originates from the tubercle of the trapezium and transverse carpal ligament, passing radially to the tendon of the flexor pollicis longus. Its tendon inserts on the radial base of the thumb proximal phalanx. Embedded in the tendon is the radial sesamoid bone. The smaller deep head arises from the trapezoid, capitate, and from the volar ligaments of the distal carpal row. The deep head of the FPB passes deep to the tendon of the flexor pollicis longus to insert onto the radial sesamoid and the base of the proximal phalanx.[13–15,17–19] An expansion of the tendon inserts onto the dorsal apparatus of the thumb.[4] The recurrent motor branch of the median nerve crosses the FPB. The vascular supply of the muscle is from the superficial palmar branch of the radial artery and from branches of the princeps pollicis and radialis indicis arteries.[10,13–15]

Innervation of the FPB can be quite variable. Both heads of the muscle may be innervated by either the median or ulnar nerve, both heads may be innervated by the median nerve alone or by the ulnar nerve exclusively, or both heads may be dually innervated.[21,22,26,27,30] The superficial head is usually innervated by the recurrent branch of the median nerve (60%), whereas the deep head is commonly innervated by the deep motor branch of the ulnar nerve.[8] In their cadaveric dissections, Day and Napier[22] found that the superficial head was supplied by the median nerve in 24 out of 30 dissections, and that the deep head was supplied by the ulnar nerve in 21 of 24 dissections. Forrest[27] found dual innervation of the superficial head in 17 out of 25 of the hands tested electromyographically. Connections between the median and ulnar nerves have been described to account for variations in innervation patterns. The Cannieu-Riche anastomosis, or the thenar ansa, is a nerve branch between the deep motor branch of the ulnar nerve and the recurrent motor branch of the median nerve that travels radially around the tendon of the flexor pollicis longus.[21,26,30] This connection has been described as occurring in up to 77% of dissections.[30]

Anomalies of the FPB have been described, including the absence of the deep head.[22] Blending of the superficial head of the FPB with OPP has been described. In addition, Bergman and Tountas[14] have described an accessory deep head or fascicle of the FPB arising from the ulnar aspect of the thumb metacarpal that inserts onto the ulnar base of the proximal phalanx.

The primary action of the FPB is to flex the thumb MCPJ. Additional actions include extension of the distal phalanx and pronation of the thumb metacarpal.[9,16–18]

The ADD

Adducere is the Latin derivation of the term adductor; its meaning is "to draw toward" (see **Figs. 2–4; Fig. 5**, see **Table 1**).[10–12] The ADD consists of two heads, an oblique and transverse head. The oblique head originates from the capitate, the bases of the second and third metacarpals, the volar intercarpal ligaments, and the sheath of the flexor carpi radialis tendon. Most of the fibers

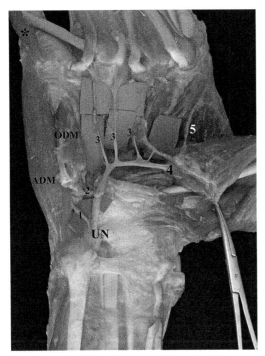

Fig. 5. Course of the deep motor branch of the ulnar nerve (UN). Motor innervation includes (1) abductor digiti minimi (ADM), flexor digiti minimi (*asterisk*), opponens digiti minimi (ODM); (3) interossei muscles; (4) ADD muscle (reflected proximally) and FPB muscle (not shown); and (5) first dorsal interosseous muscle. (*From* Leversedge F, Goldfarb C, Boyer M. Neuroanatomy. In: A pocket manual of hand and upper extremity primus manus. Philadelphia: Wolters Kluwer Lippincott Williams & Wilkins; 2010. p. 97; with permission.)

converge to unite with the tendons of the FPB (deep head) and the transverse head of the ADD to insert on the ulnar base of the thumb proximal phalanx and the dorsal extensor apparatus. A sesamoid bone is present in the tendon.[10,13,15–19] A second group of fibers coalesce beneath the tendon of the flexor pollicis longus to join the FPB (deep head) and abductor pollicis brevis. This second group of fibers has been called the "deep head" of the FPB.[13] The ADD transverse head is a triangular muscle arising from a broad base, from the distal two-thirds of the volar base of the third metacarpal. Its fibers join to insert, with the FPB and ADD oblique head, on the ulnar side of the base of the thumb proximal phalanx.[10,13]

The deep palmer arch and the deep motor branch of the ulnar nerve pass between the two heads of the ADD muscle.[10,13,15–19] The first dorsal interosseous muscle lays on the dorsum of the ADD and, together, these two muscles provide the mass of the first web space.[13] Volarly, the muscle is crossed by the index finger flexor

tendons and the first lumbrical. The princeps pollicis, radialis indicis arteries (occasionally combined as the first palmer metacarpal artery), and branches from the deep palmar arch provide the blood supply for the ADD.[13–15]

The ADD is primarily innervated by the deep motor branch of the ulnar nerve (see **Fig. 5**). Rowntree[21] demonstrated that in 2% of cases all the thenar muscles, including the ADD, were innervated only by the median nerve.

The ADD's primary action is adduction of the thumb metacarpal. The muscle also extends the thumb interphalangeal joint via its insertion onto the dorsal apparatus of the thumb.

SUMMARY

The functional mobility of the thumb, especially in its action of opposition, is a uniquely human quality. The mobility, strength, and function of the thumb are greatly affected by the actions of the intrinsic muscles of the thumb. These highly specialized muscles, with their variable innervation patterns, help to make the human hand one of the true wonders of the natural world.

ACKNOWLEDGMENTS

Special thanks to Dr Steven Green for his valuable insight.

REFERENCES

1. Bell C. The hand. Its mechanism and vital endowments as evincing design. London: William Pickering; 1833. p. 107–8.
2. Kaplan EB, Spinner M. The hand as organ. In: Spinner M, editor. Kaplan's functional and surgical anatomy of the hand. 3rd edition. Philadelphia: J.B. Lippincott; 1984. p. 3–19.
3. Austin NM. The wrist and hand complex. In: Levangie PK, Norkin CC, editors. Joint structure and function: a comprehensive analysis. 4th edition. Philadelphia: F.A. Davis Co; 2005. p. 588.
4. Kaplan EB, Riordan DC. The thumb. In: Spinner M, editor. Kaplan's functional and surgical anatomy of the hand. 3rd edition. Philadelphia: J.B. Lippincott; 1984. p. 113–51.
5. Bunnell S. Intrinsic muscles of the thumb, opposition of the thumb. In: Surgery of the Hand. Philadelphia: JB Lippincott Co; 1944. p. 388.
6. Jacobson MD, Raab R, Fazeli BM, et al. Architectural design of the human intrinsic hand muscles. J Hand Surg Am 1992;17:804–9.
7. Fahrer M. The thenar eminence: an introduction. In: Tubiana R, editor. The hand. Philadelphia: W.B. Saunders; 1981. p. 255–8.

8. Beasley RW. Surgical anatomy of the hand. In: Beasley's surgery of the hand. New York: Thieme; 2003. p. 18.

9. Kaplan EB, Smith RJ. Kinesiology of the hand and wrist and muscular variations of the hand and forearm. In: Spinner M, editor. Kaplan's functional and surgical anatomy of the hand. 3rd edition. Philadelphia: J.B. Lippincott; 1984. p. 283–349.

10. Botte MJ. Muscle anatomy. In: Doyle JR, Botte MJ, editors. Surgical anatomy of the hand and upper extremity. Philadelphia: Lippincott Williams & Wilkins; 2003. p. 149–55.

11. Dorland's Illustrated Medical Dictionary. William Alexander Newman Dorland. 31st edition. Philadelphia: WB Saunders; 2007.

12. Stedman's Medical Dictionary. Thomas Lathrop Stedman. 28th edition. Philadelphia: Lippincott Williams & Wilkins; 2006.

13. Standring S, editor. Gray's anatomy. 40th edtion. Elsevier limited; 2008.

14. Hand: Intrinsic muscles. In: Tountas CP, Bergman RA, editors. Anatomic variations of the upper etremity. New York: Churchill Livingstone Inc; 1993. p. 159–69.

15. Schmidt HM, Lanz U. Thumb. In: Surgical anatomy of the hand. Stuttgart (Germany): Georg Thieme Verlag; 2004. p. 85–113.

16. Morris's human anatomy, Part II: A complete systematic treatise by English and American authors. 4th edition. Philadelphia: P. Blakiston's Son & Co; 1907. p. 395–8. *Book digitized by Google from the library of Harvard University and uploaded to the Internet Archive.

17. Leversedge FJ. Anatomy and pathomechanics of the thumb. Hand Clin 2008;28(4):681–4.

18. Leversedge F, Goldfarb C, Boyer M. Chapter 1, Hand; Chapter 5, Neuroanatomy. In: A pocket manual of hand and upper extremity primus manus.

Philadelphia: Wolters Kluwer Lippincott Williams & Wilkins; 2010. p. 24–9, 97.

19. April EW. Hand. In: NMS clinical anatomy. 3rd edition. New York: William and Willkins; 1997. p. 109–15.

20. McFarlane RM. Observations on the functional anatomy of the intrinsic muscles of the thumb. J Bone Joint Surg Am 1962;44:1073–88.

21. Rowntree T. Anomalous innervation of the hand muscles. J Bone Joint Surg Br 1949;31(4):505–10.

22. Day MH, Napier JR. The two heads of flexor poliicis brevis. J Anat 1961;95:123–30.

23. Olave E, Prates JC, Del Sol M, et al. Distribution patterns of the muscular branch of the median nerve in the thenar region. J Anat 1995;186:441–6.

24. Mumford J, Morecraft R, Blair WF. Anatomy of the thenar branch of the median nerve. J Hand Surg Am 1987;12(3):361–5.

25. Littler JW. Tendon transfers and arthrodesis in combined median and ulnar nerve paralysis. J Bone Joint Surg Am 1949;31(2):225–34.

26. Ajmani ML. Variations in the motor nerve supply of the thenar and hypothenar muscles of the hand. J Anat 1996;189(Pt 1):145–50.

27. Forrest WJ. Motor innervation of human thenar and hypothenar muscles in 25 hands: a study combining electromyography and percutaneous nerve stimulation. Can J Surg 1967;10(2):196–9.

28. Harness D, Sekeles E, Chaco J. The double innervation of the opponens pollicis muscle: an electromyographic study. J Anat 1974;117(Pt 2):329–31.

29. Kapandji IA. Biomechanics of the thumb. In: Tubiana R, editor. The hand. Philadelphia: W.B. Saunders; 1981. p. 404–22.

30. Harness D, Sekeles E. The double anastomotic innervation of thenar muscles. J Anat 1971;109(Pt 3):461–6.

dynamic movements. Interosseous muscle action and static posture seem to be the "foundation" for all practical and efficient hand function against which the extrinsic flexors and extensors are balanced.

The conjoined insertions of the interossei into the bone of the proximal phalanges *and* the extensor aponeurosis give these muscles antagonistic advantage in balancing the larger excursions of the extrinsic flexors and extensors of the digits, therefore optimizing the action of integrated finger flexion and extension. Rules often have exceptions, however, and as Brand and Hollister[1] pointed out in summarizing the findings of Salisbury, variability of the dorsal interossei insertions raises (but does not answer) the question as to whether the lumbricals may act in lieu of the dorsal interossei in those cases where the dorsal interossei have no insertion into the extensor hood.

An illustrative example of the interosseous muscles' *typical* effects on hand function can be made by comparison to the hydraulics of a backhoe: the hydraulics that stabilize the backhoe arm at its base (or the weight of its carrying load) and keep it from falling forward or backward, are analogous to the interossei. Balanced against this foundation, the backhoe arm is able to be positioned for functional delivery of loads and delicate movements of its bucket by its other "extrinsic hydraulics." Without the "intrinsic hydraulic" stability, the backhoe arm, or even the entire structure, would topple.

It is also important to define and understand the fascial boundaries of the interosseous muscles, as compartment syndrome can and does occur within the "interosseous space." There are both palmar and dorsal layers of incorporating fascia that enclose all the interosseous muscles and the finger metacarpals. Emanuel Kaplan[2] and subsequently many other authors[3] include the adductor pollicis muscle as being incorporated by the contiguous fascial layers with the interossei and therefore consider it as part of the interosseous compartment (see **Fig. 1**E).

The relative contributions that the interossei make to composite grip and pinch strength has been reported in the literature, and are pivotal to understanding both normal and pathologic hand function. Kozin and colleagues[4] demonstrated an overall decrease in grip strength of 38% and 77% decrease in key pinch by measuring them after ulnar nerve block in healthy individuals. This simple yet instructive study suggests a critical contribution by the interossei to key pinch. The study also demonstrated that each median and ulnar innervated musculature had about a 40% contribution to overall grip strength, the implication being that the balance can be, to a large degree, attributable to the extrinsics.

The relative contributions of the interossei and the lumbricals to IP extension and MP flexion have been discussed and are relevant to understanding the effects and treatment of nerve palsies in the hand. Lumbrical action is discussed in the article by Vigler and Palti elsewhere in this issue. Although both muscle groups act in concert, Eyler and Markee[5] explained that the volar interossei are strong IP joint extensors throughout the arc of MP flexion, whereas the lumbricals lose effectiveness in this function as MP flexion increases. Although both the volar and dorsal interossei contribute significantly to MP flexion force throughout the entire arc of MP flexion, it appears that the lumbricals give their maximum contribution to MP flexion force closer to terminal MP flexion, especially in the case of the index finger. Valentin[6] further subcategorized the interosseous contributions to IP extension and MP flexion as variable based on the presence or absence of their insertion into the extensor hood, but acknowledged that these were exceptions to the rule. These anatomic variances nonetheless can manifest with paradoxic hand function and posture in nerve palsies, and are therefore worthy of consideration.

PATHOLOGIC FUNCTION

High and low ulnar nerve palsy, ischemic contracture, postfracture/crush injury loss of muscle compliance, median nerve palsy, and improper splinting and cast positioning can all lead to failure of function of the interosseous muscles. The removal or impairment of the interosseous functional forces, whether by static contracture or loss of dynamic contraction, results in an imbalance in integrated finger function and loss of grip and pinch strength.

In the case of failure of dynamic action of the interossei, such as is the case with ulnar nerve injury and in the special case of median nerve injury (See the article by Vigler and Palti elsewhere in this issue for further exploration of this topic), the resultant interruption of finger balance leads to an "intrinsic minus" deformity, with MP joint hyperextension, and both PIP and DIP joint flexion. This is because the interossei are the principal flexors of the MP joints and extensors of the PIP joints, whereas the extrinsic extensors are not strong PIP extensors. Furthermore, the slackening of the axial tension on the interosseous insertion into the extensor aponeurosis diminishes the normal DIP extension force of its oblique retinacular ligaments, and the overpull of the flexor profundus muscles results in DIP flexion deformity.

Chronic unattended ulnar palsy also leads to progressive insufficiency of the MP joint volar plates and the eventual hyperextension contracture seen in both high and low nerve deficits.

Ischemic insults (compartment syndrome), severe swelling, inappropriate or prolonged casting and splinting, and delays in and ineffective hand therapy can lead to contracture of the interossei and a stiff hand and fingers in ulnar plus *or* ulnar minus position. Although the effects of ischemia are in many instances beyond control, improper positioning of hand splints and casts, and timing of hand therapy clearly are manageable. The optimal position for splinting and casting the hand and wrist keeps the MP joints flexed approximately 60° and leaves the PIP joints free to be moved through flexion and extension to allow for interosseous stretching. Certainly, the effect of immobilization on the interosseous muscles is not the first consideration in choosing methods of fixation for hand and finger fractures, but should be considered in the context of early postoperative movement (or the effects of limitations of movement) in every case.

SUMMARY

The delicate balance of integrated finger function is rooted in both dynamic and isometric actions of the interosseous muscles. Although the origins of the palmar and dorsal groups distinguish each group with the different actions of adduction and abduction of the fingers, respectively, perhaps even more critical to hand function are the synergistic effects both groups have in working as intrinsic MP flexors and PIP extensors, and the antagonistic effects on extrinsic flexors and extensors. Denervation of the interosseous muscles causes intrinsic minus deformity and interruption of integrated finger flexion function as well as substantial deficit in pinch strength. Loss of movement, resulting from paralysis of these muscles, can manifest as contracture and hand dysfunction in any position. An understanding of interosseous muscle compartment anatomy and function, therefore, is essential to identifying compartment syndrome, choosing appropriate treatment modalities, and avoiding pitfalls of postinjury recovery across the entire spectrum of pathologic conditions of the hand and fingers.

REFERENCES

1. Brand PW, Hollister AM. Clinical mechanics of the hand. 3rd edition. St Louis (MO): Mosby; 1999.
2. Kaplan EB. Functional and surgical anatomy of the hand. Philadelphia: Lippincott; 1953.
3. Schreuders TA, Brandsma JW, Stam HJ. The intrinsic muscles of the hand. Phys Med Rehab Kuror 2006; 16:1–9.
4. Kozin SH, Porter S, Clark P, et al. The contribution of the intrinsic muscles to grip and pinch strength. J Hand Surg Am 1999;24(1):64–72.
5. Eyler DL, Markee JE. The anatomy and function of the intrinsic musculature of the fingers. J Bone Joint Surg Am 1954;36:1–10.
6. Valentin P. The interossei and the lumbricals. chapters 24 and 25. In: Tubiana R, editor, The hand, vol. 1. Philadelphia: WB Saunders; 1981. p. 244–50.

Anatomy and Function of Lumbrical Muscles

Ram Palti, MD[a], Mordechai Vigler, MD[b],*

KEYWORDS

- Lumbricals • Intrinsics • Extensor mechanism

The lumbricals (Latin for worm) are worm-shaped muscles of the palm that are unique in that they arise on their antagonist and their origin and main insertion are tendons: the flexor digitorum profundus (FDP) and the extensor expansion, respectively. The lumbricals assist in metacarpophalangeal joint flexion; they contribute to interphalangeal joint extension by acting as deflexors of the proximal interphalangeal joint.

ANATOMY

The 4 cylindrical lumbrical muscles are located in the midpalm, dorsal to the palmar aponeurosis. The muscles have a movable origin, arising from the tendons of the FDP muscles, their almost parallel fibers course distally, palmar to the transverse intermetacarpal ligaments, and insert on the radial side of the digits. In the most common pattern of origin, the first and second lumbricals originate from the radial side of the first and second deep flexors; the third and fourth lumbricals originate from bipennate muscle bellies on the adjacent surfaces of the FDP tendons.[1,2] Many anatomic variants of the lumbrical origins are described, which differ in the number of double-headed (bipennate) lumbricals and the proximity of the origin.[2–5] For example, the first lumbrical in most cases has 1 radial head, although variations include an additional head either from the flexor pollicis longus (FPL), FDP, or flexor digitorum superficialis (FDS) of the middle digit.[2] These muscles tend to follow a pattern of increasing variability from the radial to the ulnar side; the third and fourth lumbricals show the highest rate of variability in origin.

Zancolli[6] and Smith[7] described the lumbricals as contributing only to the lateral band mechanism. More recent cadaver studies suggest that the lumbricals have variable insertions: proximal phalanx, volar plate of the metacarpophalangeal joint, and extensor apparatus (lateral band, transverse and oblique fibers of the extensor hood). Although all lumbricals attach to the lateral band, extra insertions either on the oblique fibers or the transverse fibers or both were found in up to 58% muscles dissected. Up to 48% of lumbricals have volar plate and/or bony attachments. Only 25% of muscles insert exclusively to the radial lateral band.[5] Extra insertions to the extensor mechanism are more common with the first lumbrical and attachments to bone and volar plate are most frequent with the fourth lumbrical.[5,8] The higher rate of variability found in both origins and insertions of the ulnar-sided lumbricals may explain the most common presentation of camptodactyly at the little and ring digits.

The lumbrical muscles are highly specialized in terms of architectural properties. Their muscle mass and physiologic cross-sectional area are lowest in the upper extremity, whereas the ratio between fiber and muscle length is largest in the upper limb. This pattern indicates that the lumbricals are designed for high excursions and that the muscle contractile force is constant over a wide range of fiber lengths, depending on the position of the FDP tendon.[3]

The first and second lumbricals are always innervated by the median nerve, whereas the third and forth lumbricals are usually innervated by the ulnar nerve. However, in 25%, the third lumbrical might be innervated by the median rather than

The authors have nothing to disclose.

[a] Department of Hand Surgery, Sheba Medical Center, Ramat Gan, Israel
[b] Department of Orthopaedic Surgery, Rabin Medical Center, Hasharon Hospital, 17A Ha'atzmaut Street, Petach-Tikva 49379, Israel
* Corresponding author.
E-mail address: drvigler@gmail.com

Hand Clin 28 (2012) 13–17
doi:10.1016/j.hcl.2011.09.002

the ulnar nerve.[9] The first lumbrical is innervated through the radial digital nerve to the index digit, whereas the second lumbrical is innervated by the corresponding common digital nerve to the index and middle digits.[8,10] The finding that innervation of the first 2 lumbricals arises from the digital nerves indicates that the digital nerves are not purely sensory and it is prudent to protect the innervations of the lumbricals during mobilization of the digital nerves.

Each of the 2 medial lumbricals is supplied by a single and separate branch from the deep branch of the ulnar nerve. Although the ulnar nerve branching varies, the branches to the lumbricals are comparatively long and partially enveloped in mobile fascia to enable smooth motion of the muscles.[11]

Innervation of the lumbricals occurs typically in the proximal to middle third junctions of the muscle. In the transverse plane, the nerve invariably enters the first 2 lumbricals in the radial-palmar aspect, and the third and fourth lumbricals in the ulnar-dorsal aspect.[8,10,11] Diameters of the nerves innervating the lumbricals range from 0.30 to 1.86 mm, with a mean of 1.17 mm.

The vascular supply to the lumbricals is from 4 different sources: superficial palmar arch (SPA), common digital arteries, deep palmar arch and palmar metacarpal arteries, and dorsal digital arteries.[4,12] The main blood supply of these muscles is the SPA. Each of the lumbricals has a segmental blood supply and receives blood from both its palmar and dorsal surfaces. There are considerable variations in topography of the principal branches in different lumbrical muscles, but the vascular supply of the first and second lumbricals is more consistent and enters their proximal portion. Hence, when considering the use of the lumbricals as a proximally based axial pedicle flap, the 2 radial lumbricals are more appropriate than the ulnar ones because of their size, comparatively fewer variations in origin, and their vascular and nerve supply.[4,8]

Lumbrical Function

The lumbrical muscle is the workhorse of the extensor apparatus.[7] Electromyography of the lumbrical reveals high levels of activity whenever there is active extension of the interphalangeal joints. Strong electrical stimulation of the lumbrical produces interphalangeal joint extension followed by metacarpophalangeal joint flexion. Low levels of electric stimulation produce only interphalangeal joint extension. There is no radial deviation of the digit when the lumbrical contracts.[7]

Because the lumbrical arises from the FDP tendon, it is the only muscle that is able to relax the tendon of its antagonist. When considering lumbrical action, it is best to consider its 2 attachments: to the profundus tendon and to the lateral band. Thus, if the profundus contracts and the lumbrical relaxes, the interphalangeal joints of the digits flex. If the profundus is relaxed, contraction of the lumbrical pulls the lateral band proximally and the profundus tendon distally. The viscoelastic force provided by the profundus tendon within the digit is lessened and the interphalangeal joints fully extend. The lumbrical thus contributes to interphalangeal joint extension by decreasing the flexor torque.[13] When both the profundus and the lumbrical contract, the interphalangeal joints and metacarpophalangeal joint flex simultaneously.

Flexion of the proximal phalanx is achieved chiefly by the interossei because electromyography has indicated that, in normal circumstances, the lumbrical contributes little to metacarpophalangeal joint flexion. Buford and colleagues[14] showed that the lumbrical contributes only 2% of the overall flexion moment at the index metacarpophalangeal joint. However, when the interossei are paralyzed, the lumbrical can initiate flexion at this joint. Ranney and colleagues[15] showed that the lumbrical acting alone can flex the metacarpophalangeal joint. Using a cadaver hand, isolated lumbrical contraction was mechanically simulated, acting against a spring model of the index extrinsic muscles. Flexion of the proximal phalanx may also be achieved through contraction of the FDS and profundus. When these muscles contract, they first flex the interphalangeal joints. After full interphalangeal joint flexion is achieved, the long flexors flex the metacarpophalangeal joint until the digit is completely closed. If digit flexion were solely performed by the FDP and superficialis, metacarpophalangeal joint flexion would occur only after interphalangeal joint flexion were complete, as seen in palsy of the intrinsics.

The lumbrical has the smallest physiologic cross-sectional area of the intrinsic muscles. It is not a strong muscle. However lumbrical muscle fibers extend 85% to 90% of the muscle length, indicating that the lumbrical is designed for large excursions. This suggestion has been confirmed by Jacobson and colleagues,[3] who showed that, of the 45 muscles in the human upper limb, the lumbrical had the highest fiber length (FL)/muscle length (ML) ratio. The high FL/ML ratio results in a flatter, broader length-tension curve that allows constant contractile force over a long range of fiber lengths, depending on the position of the FDP tendon. It is thought that long lumbrical muscle fiber length (average 40–48 mm) might facilitate active muscle contraction, even during

FDP contraction, by allowing the lumbrical origin to move without large changes in sarcomere length.[3] With a short lumbrical fiber length, FDP excursion could stretch the lumbrical sarcomeres to a point at which they would be unable to generate active force.[3]

The lumbrical muscles are richly endowed with muscle spindles. Their passive elongation by contraction of the FDP may inhibit digit extensors and facilitate wrist extensors.[13,14,16,17] For this reason, the lumbrical muscles have been called tensionmeters between the flexors and extensors.[18] Leijnse and Kalker[19] concluded that the lumbricals are in the optimal position for proprioceptive feedback regarding proximal interphalangeal–distal interphalangeal joint motion. The unique properties of the lumbricals indicate that they are probably important in fast, alternating movements, such as typing and playing instruments.[20]

Strength

Manual muscle strength testing of the lumbricals is difficult because of the synergistic action of the interosseous muscles. Schreuders and Stam[21] showed that, in patients with ulnar nerve paralysis (nonfunctioning interosseous muscles), the strength of the lumbrical muscles in the index and long digits (as measured by metacarpophalangeal joint flexion strength) was only 12% of the strength of the noninvolved hand.[21,22]

From a therapy point of view, there is no specific exercise program for strengthening the lumbrical muscles. Strength training is similar to interosseous muscle training, with perhaps more focus on speed and coordination.

Relationship of Thumb to Fingers: Why the Thumb is Devoid of a Lumbrical

The thumb has a highly mobile carpometacarpal joint but lacks a middle phalanx. Therefore, it has no proximal interphalangeal joint and consequently no mechanical need for a lumbrical. Because the thumb has excellent coordination without a lumbrical, the function of the lumbrical as a sense organ cannot be simply to coordinate finger movement.

Lumbricals arise from the tendons of the flexor profundus muscle and are supplied by the same nerves, even sharing the division of nerve fibers into median and ulnar nerves. It is therefore appropriate to consider the lumbricals as flexors of the fingers, even though they act to aid extension at the interphalangeal joints. By contracting, they unload the larger of 2 passive flexor forces. Therefore, on being passively stretched, it is speculated that they inhibit the extensors of the fingers, and

this facilitates progressive flexion of all joints in this long chain of articulations on concentric contraction of the FDP. Because there is an extra joint in the finger that the thumb does not possess, an extra flexor, the superficial flexor, is needed in the finger, and with it a hybrid type of flexor-extensor, the lumbrical.[23]

Movement of some digits may or may not be restricted by that of adjacent digits. The thumb is completely free, followed in order of decreasing independence by the index, little, middle, and ring fingers. Restrictions in freedom of movement of the finger occurs in the medial 3 fingers because of interconnection of the junctura tendinei of the extensor digitorum. The ring finger is the most restricted because it lies between the other two. Simply dividing these connections makes no difference because there are muscular interconnections on the flexor side. The third and fourth lumbrical muscles each arise from 2 profundus tendons and, in this way, the 3 profundus tendons are bound together. In addition, these 3 profundus tendons share a common muscle belly on the flexor side and also a common antagonist on the extensor side. The lack of independence is therefore caused by a combination of both junctures and lumbricals.

LUMBRICAL-PLUS FINGER

There is a delicate balance between the tendon of the FDP and the lumbrical muscle. If the tendon of the profundus is lacerated within the digit, the normal tone of the profundus muscle belly pulls its cut end and the attachment of the lumbrical proximally. The retracted lumbrical causes increased tension on the radial lateral band, and the proximal interphalangeal joint may extend or hyperextend when the finger is actively flexed. This paradoxic extension is known as the lumbrical-plus finger.[7] Distal amputation, which severs the profundus tendon, can produce comparable consequences.

If a flexor tendon graft is inserted too loosely, a lumbrical-plus finger will result. When the patient tries to flex the interphalangeal joints, the contracting profundus pulls first on the lumbrical rather than on the loose tendon graft, producing paradoxic extension of the proximal interphalangeal joint. Occasionally, a lumbrical belly is wrapped about the site of the tendon juncture in a tendon graft. If the muscle fibers become ischemic or tight, a lumbrical-plus finger may also result.

Relationship of Lumbricals to Carpal Tunnel Syndrome

Carpal tunnel syndrome is usually caused by thickened flexor tenosynovium that compresses the median nerve.

Several reports have suggested that anomalous proximal muscle origins or hypertrophy of the lumbrical muscles may also cause this compressive neuropathy.[24–29] If the lumbrical muscles were to originate proximal to the transverse carpal ligament, hypertrophy (secondary to repetitive use) could contribute to compression of the median nerve.[30–35] Cobb and colleagues[36,37] concluded that lumbrical muscle incursion into the carpal tunnel can result in increase of carpal tunnel pressure in cadaver hands and could be a variable in the cause of work-related carpal tunnel syndrome. Siegal and colleagues,[38] as well as Mehta and Gardner,[39] showed in cadaveric dissections that the lumbrical muscles originate distal to the carpal canal with the fingers held in the extended position. Siegal and colleagues[38] also showed that all 4 lumbrical muscles lie within the carpal canal when the fingers are actively flexed by proximal retraction of the FDP tendons.

Other causes of carpal tunnel syndrome with respect to the lumbricals include anatomic variants such as abnormally long lumbrical muscles[28] and aberrant tendinous origin of the first lumbrical.[24] An anomalous origin of the lumbrical from the FDP has the potential to cause compression of the median nerve in the carpal tunnel.[40]

Sparing of the innervation to the lumbrical muscles in carpal tunnel syndrome has been attributed to the funicular position of the lumbrical motor axons within the median nerve in the wrist. The branches to the lumbricals are more dorsal and therefore better protected from direct compression.[41]

SUMMARY

The lumbrical muscles are unique in having their origin and insertion on tendons. Anatomically, they are highly specialized in terms of their architectural properties, with a small physiologic cross-sectional area but long fiber length. Their unique properties indicate that they are probably important in fast, alternating movements and fine-tuning digit motion.

REFERENCES

1. Shin YA, Amadio PC. Stiff finger joints. In: Green's operative hand surgery. 5th edition. Philadelphia: Elsevier; 2005. p. 422–3.
2. Goldberg S. The origin of the lumbrical muscles in the hand of the South African native. Hand 1970;2: 168–71.
3. Jacobson MD, Raab R, Fazeli BM, et al. Architectural design of the human intrinsic hand muscles. J Hand Surg Am 1992;17:804–9.
4. Okan B, Pinar Y, Ozer MA, et al. The vascular anatomy of the lumbrical muscles in the hand. J Plast Reconstr Aesthet Surg 2007;60(10):1120–6.
5. Eladoumikdachi F, Valkov PL, Thomas J, et al. Anatomy of the intrinsic hand muscles revisited: part II. Lumbricals. Plast Reconstr Surg 2002; 110(5):1225–31.
6. Zancolli EA. Structural and dynamic bases of hand surgery. 2nd edition. Philadelphia: Lippincott; 1979.
7. Smith RJ. Intrinsic muscles of the fingers: function, dysfunction and surgical reconstruction. In: AAOS instructional course lectures, vol. 24. St Louis (MO): Mosby; 1975. p. 200–20.
8. Koncilia H, Kuzbari R, Worseg A, et al. The lumbrical muscle flap: anatomic study and clinical application. J Hand Surg 1998;23:111–9.
9. Sunderland S, Ray LJ. Metrical and non metrical features of the muscular branches of the median nerve. J Comp Neurol 1946;85:191–201.
10. Lauritzen RS, Szabo RM. Innervation of the lumbrical muscles. J Hand Surg 1996;21:57–8.
11. Atkins SE, Logan B, McGrouther DA. The deep (motor) branch of the ulnar nerve: a detailed examination of its course and the clinical significance of its damage. J Hand Surg Eur Vol 2009;34:47–57.
12. Zbrodowski A, Mariéthoz E, Bednarkiewicz M, et al. The blood supply of the lumbrical muscles. J Hand Surg 1998;23:384–8.
13. Ranney D, Wells R. Lumbrical muscle function as revealed by a new and physiological approach. Anat Rec 1988;222(1):110–4.
14. Buford WL Jr, Koh S, Andersen CR, et al. Analysis of intrinsic-extrinsic muscle function through interactive 3-dimensional kinematic simulation and cadaver studies. J Hand Surg Am 2005;30(6):1267–75.
15. Ranney DA, Wells RP, Dowling J. Lumbrical function: interaction of lumbrical contraction with the elasticity of the extrinsic finger muscles and its effect on metacarpophalangeal equilibrium. J Hand Surg Am 1987;12(4):566–75.
16. Backhouse KM, Catton WT. An experimental study of the function of the lumbrical muscles in the human hand. J Anat 1954;88(5):133–41.
17. Devanadan MS, Ghosh S, John KL. A quantitative study of the muscle spindles and tendon organs in some intrinsic muscles of the hand. Anat Rec 1983;207:263–6.
18. Rabischong P. Basic problems in the restoration of prehension. Ann Chir 1971;25(19):927–33.
19. Leijnse JN, Kalker JJ. A two-dimensional kinematic model of the lumbrical in the human finger. J Biomech 1995;28(3):237–49.
20. Leijnse JN. Why the lumbrical muscle should not be bigger – a force model of the lumbrical in the unloaded human finger. J Biomech 1997;30(11–12): 1107–14.

21. Schreuders TA, Stam HJ. Strength measurements of the lumbrical muscles. J Hand Ther 1996;9(4):303–5.

22. Schreuders TA, Brandsma JW, Stam HJ. The intrinsic muscles of the hand. Phys Med Rehab Kuror 2006; 16:1–9.

23. Ranney D. The hand as a concept: digital differences and their importance. Clin Anat 1995;8:281–7.

24. Butler B Jr, Bigley EC Jr. Aberrant index lumbrical tendinous origin associated with carpal tunnel syndrome: a case report. J Bone Joint Surg 1971;53:160–2.

25. Schultz RJ, Endler PM, Huddleston HD. Anomalous median nerve and an anomalous muscle belly of the first lumbrical associated with carpal tunnel syndrome. J Bone Joint Surg 1973;55:1744–6.

26. Still JM Jr, Kleinert HE. Anomalous muscles and nerve entrapment in the wrist and hand. Plast Reconsrt Surg 1973;52:394–400.

27. Jabaley ME. Personal observations on the role of the lumbrical muscles in carpal tunnel syndrome. J Hand Surg 1978;3:82–4.

28. Erikson J. A case of carpal tunnel syndrome on the basis of abnormally long lumbrical muscle. Acta Orthop Scand 1973;44:275–7.

29. Robinson D, Aghasi M, Halperin N. The treatment of carpal tunnel syndrome caused by hypertrophied lumbrical muscles. Scand J Plast Reconstr Surg 1989;23:149–51.

30. Gainer JV, Nugent GR. Carpal tunnel syndrome: report of 430 operations. South Med J 1977;70:325–8.

31. Rothfleisch S, Sherman D. Carpal tunnel syndrome, biomechanical aspects of occupational occurrence and implications regarding surgical management. Orthop Rev 1978;7:107–9.

32. Smith EM, Sonstegard DA, Anderson WH Jr. Carpal tunnel syndrome: contribution of flexor tendons. Arch Phys Med Rehabil 1977;58:379–85.

33. Nissen K. Tunnel tactics. BMJ 1974;3:624.

34. Gelberman RH, Hergenroeder PT, Hargens AA, et al. The carpal tunnel syndrome: a study of canal pressures. J Bone Joint Surg 1981;63:380–3.

35. Skie M, Zeiss J, Ebraheim NA, et al. Carpal tunnel changes and median nerve compression during wrist flexion and extension seen by magnetic resonance imaging. J Hand Surg 1990;15:934–9.

36. Cobb TK, An KN, Cooney WP. Effect of lumbrical muscle incursion within the carpal tunnel on carpal tunnel pressure: a cadaveric study. J Hand Surg Am 1995;20(2):186–92.

37. Cobb TK, An KN, Cooney WP, et al. Lumbrical muscle incursion into the carpal tunnel during finger flexion. J Hand Surg Br 1994;19(4):434–8.

38. Siegel DB, Tucson AZ, Kuzma G, et al. Anatomic investigation of the role of the lumbrical muscles in carpal tunnel syndrome. J Hand Surg Am 1995;20: 860–3.

39. Mehta HJ, Gardner WU. A study of lumbrical muscles in the human hand. Am J Anat 1961;109: 227–38.

40. Goto S, Kojima T. An anomalous lumbrical muscle with an independent muscle belly associated with carpal tunnel syndrome. Handchir Mikochir Plast Chir 1993;25(2):72–4.

41. Yates SK, Yaworski R, Brown WF. Relative preservation of lumbrical versus thenar motor fibres in neurogenic disorders. J Neurol Neurosurg Psychiatry 1981;44(9):768–74.

Anatomy and Function of the Hypothenar Muscles

John A. Pasquella, DO[a],*, Pam Levine, MD[b]

KEYWORDS

- Anatomy • Function • Hypothenar
- Muscle • Hand • Intrinsic

The hypothenar eminence is the thick soft tissue mass located on the ulnar side of the palm. Understanding its location and contents is important for understanding certain aspects of hand function. The hypothenar eminence is located palmar to the hamate, pisiform, fifth metacarpal bones and the proximal portion of the fifth finger proximal phalanx. The hypothenar eminence comprises the pisotriquetral complex, Guyon canal, and hypothenar space.[1]

The pisotriquetral complex is formed of the flexor and extensor retinaculum, flexor carpi ulnaris (FCU) tendon, triangular fibrocartilage complex, pisohamate ligament, pisometacarpal ligament, and the abductor digiti minimi (ADM) muscle, which is one of the hypothenar muscles. The function of the pisotriquetral complex is to provide stability to the pisotriquetral joint, which is important in ulnar-sided wrist kinematics.[2]

The Guyon canal (also known as the ulnar tunnel) is located on the anteromedial aspect of the wrist. Within its canal traverses the ulnar neurovascular bundle as it passes from the forearm into the palm. It is important to understand that the canal is not a rigid structure but varies in its dimensions from the proximal to distal aspects.[1] Understanding the anatomy of Guyon's canal is important because the hypothenar muscles contribute to the structure of the canal.

The medial (or ulnar) wall of the canal comprises the pisiform, FCU, and ADM. The lateral wall is made up of the transverse carpal ligament (TCL),

hook of the hamate, and the flexor digiti minimi (FDM). The roof is formed of the palmaris brevis muscle and volar carpal ligament, whereas the floor is formed of the TCL, pisohamate ligament, pisometacarpal ligament, and opponens digiti minimi (ODM).[3] The importance of the canal regarding the hypothenar muscles becomes evident later during the discussion on nerve innervation.

The final component of the eminence is the hypothenar space. There are a total of 3 spaces in the hand: the hypothenar space, thenar space, and midcarpal space. The hypothenar space differs from the other spaces in that there are no extrinsic flexor tendons that pass through it. Instead, it is made up of the 3 hypothenar muscles. These muscles are the ADM, FDM brevis, and ODM.[1]

MUSCULAR ANATOMY AND FUNCTION

The anatomic origin and insertions of the hypothenar muscles have been studied closely over the years through cadaveric dissections. It is well known that there is a large degree of variability of the hypothenar muscles even when compared with the contralateral extremity.[4]

The hypothenar muscles collectively originate partially from the TCL, volar carpal ligament, and adjacent carpal bones. Kung and colleagues[5] examined 10 fresh frozen cadaveric hands and wrists to identify the amount of the hypothenar mass that originated from the TCL. They found that 49% of the hypothenar muscle mass

The authors have nothing to disclose.
a Department of Hand Surgery, New York University Hospital for Joint Diseases Orthopaedic Institute, 301 East 17th Street, New York City, NY 10003, USA
b 35 Prospect Park West, Brooklyn, NY 11215, USA
* Corresponding author.
E-mail address: JohnP75@gmail.com

Hand Clin 28 (2012) 19–25
doi:10.1016/j.hcl.2011.09.003
0749-0712/12/$ – see front matter © 2012 Elsevier Inc. All rights reserved.

originated from the TCL, 24% from the volar carpal ligament, and the remaining 28% from the hook of the hamate and pisiform in equal distribution.[5]

There has been speculation in recent years that release of the TCL during a carpal tunnel decompression may cause altered kinematics of the ulnar-sided carpal bones. Theoretically, this change in carpal dynamics may cause a shortening of the hypothenar muscles. Many investigators have proposed that this muscle shortening could be the cause of perceived weakness in grip strength after a carpal tunnel release.[6,7]

Another anatomic study, Murata and colleagues[4] investigated variations in hypothenar muscle origin and insertion. They dissected 35 cadaveric hands to identify the muscle origins and insertions, number of muscle bellies, and any anatomic anomaly.

The ADM muscle originated from the pisiform, tendon of the FCU, and pisohamate ligament. In most of the cadaveric specimens, Murata and colleagues[4] found that the ADM had 2 muscle slips, each with a different insertion: one slip inserted into the ulnar aspect of the small finger proximal phalanx base and the other slip into the extensor apparatus of the small finger.[4] The primary function of the ADM is small finger abduction, and it also contributes to small finger metacarpophalangeal (MP) flexion and interphalangeal extension.[8]

The FDM muscle originates from the hook of the hamate, ulnar portion of the flexor retinaculum, and radial portion of the pisiform. In most cases, there is 1 muscle belly. Distally, the muscle fuses with the ADM. However, Murata and colleagues[4] did note some unusual findings. They found that the FDM was absent in 8 of the specimens. In 3 specimens, the FDM existed independently from the ADM. In these cases, the muscle inserted distally into the volar aspect of the fifth metacarpal head. The greater moment arm of the FDM is responsible for small finger MP flexion, making this the primary function. However, the FDM does contribute to small finger abduction as well.[8] This explains why the small finger maintains some abduction after an abductor digiti quinti transfer to restore thumb opposition.

The mechanical action of the FDM and ADM relies partly on the stability of the pisiform related to their attachment on this bone. The pisiform is mobile; therefore, its relative position is influenced by the action of the FCU, which envelopes the pisiform with its tendon sheath. Even though the motion of the pisiform in cadaveric studies has been shown to be within a 1.4-cm range, physiologically the motion is probably less than 0.5 cm.[8]

The ODM muscle has 2 layers with separate muscle origins. The superficial layer originates from the hook of the hamate and inserts into the distal ulnar aspect of the fifth metacarpal shaft. The deep layer originates from the ulnar flexor compartment wall adjacent to the hamate hook and inserts into the proximal ulnar aspect of the small finger metacarpal shaft.[4]

The ODM muscle lies deep to the other 2 hypothenar muscles. It is distinct from the ADM and FDM in that it is the only one that inserts into the fifth metacarpal. The combined force vector of these individual muscle layers exerts an action that flexes and opposes the fifth metacarpal. It has no attachment distal to the MP joint; thus, its sole function is to move the metacarpal.[8]

When the metacarpal is flexed by action of the hypothenar muscles, the FCU contracts to stabilize the pisiform. This mechanism causes the ulnar arch to become exaggerated in a process called cupping. In addition to maintaining the ulnar palmar arch, cupping allows the hand to perform specific functions such as holding fluids or food. This is a basic necessary function for many cultures especially in societies in which utensils are not used for eating. This is more prevalent in the Eastern societies. However, even in the Western society, loss of the ulnar palmar arch provides some functional impairment, as well as being aesthetically displeasing.[8]

There is another function of the hypothenar muscles that many would consider equally important. The 3 muscles together provide a very stout soft tissue mass on the ulnar border of the hand. This soft tissue mass can absorb forces imparted onto the hand, which allows them to disseminate that energy across many layers of muscle fibers. The ability of these muscles to function in this capacity makes them excellent shock absorbers. Other than providing a soft cushion to protect the underlying bony anatomy, they can diminish shear stress across the palm that might be felt during certain activities. Simply resting ones hand on a desk and using a stapler are functions one is capable of performing secondary to the padding provided by the hypothenar muscles. In addition, certain workers like a masseuse rely on the function of the hypothenar muscles as a soft tissue mass to perform their daily activities.[8]

Instinctively, individuals use the hypothenar eminence as a hammer to apply a blunt force to another object. For example, a person might apply this force to open a box or bang on a door. The anatomic position of the palm during these hammer thrusts has been studied. As the palm applies a blunt force to an object, the hypothenar eminence accounts for most of the contact surface area. In fact, the pisiform is the only bony structure to come into contact with the opposed object. It is able to withstand a certain amount of traumatic force because of its mobility within the FCU sheath. At no point during the hammer thrust does the underlying metacarpal make contact with the opposing surface.[9]

This function of the hypothenar eminence is best represented by the activity of a martial arts expert while engaging in hammer techniques like breaking a board or cement block. The karate chop, as investigated by Fahrer,[9] occurs when the medial side of the palm engages an object with the intent to break it. This technique is routinely performed by martial artists during training exercises, demonstrations, or competitions without injury to their hand. After careful photographic evaluation of a trained professional performing a karate chop, the position of the hand during impact was determined. In the anteroposterior view, the palm is positioned 45° toward the midline, and in the lateral view, the hypothenar eminence is positioned in about 15°. Perhaps, this position of the hypothenar eminence during impact optimizes its shock-absorbing characteristics.[9]

Dissection of the hypothenar soft tissue mass has provided valuable information in understanding the ability of this area of the palm to withstand tremendous forces. First, the skin is much thicker and more durable than the skin on the thenar surface. It resembles the skin that overlies the palmar aponeurosis. Deep to this thick palmar skin is a complex fibrous shell, which attaches firmly to the undersurface of the dermis. This fibrous shell forms a meshwork of tendinous fibers that encapsulate small lobules of fat. It is approximately 2 mm in thickness and overlies the hypothenar space. Located between the fibrous shell and the hypothenar muscular fascia is a yellow semi-fluid fat layer. This fat can move around freely; thus, it can become easily displaced when a direct force is applied to the ulnar side of the palm. The interconnection of this dense fibrous network with an underlying fat layer is one of the key characteristics of the hypothenar eminence, which makes it a great shock absorber.[9]

In addition to the anatomic variations regarding the origin and insertion of the hypothenar muscles, there are a few reported cases of anomalous muscle structures within the hypothenar space. Curry and Kuz[10] reported on a finding during dissection of a cadaveric forearm and wrist. They reported on a muscle mass deep to the superficial layer of the flexor retinaculum. The muscle originated from a tendon slip from the distal part of the palmaris longus tendon approximately 5 cm proximal to the palmar aponeurosis. The tendon slip passed distally through Guyon's canal between the ADM and FDM muscles. The distal

portion of the anomalous muscle joined the deep head of the ADM muscle, and together they inserted into the proximal phalanx. The clinical implications of this anomaly are unknown because it was an incidental finding during a routine dissection.

Failla[11] reported on 2 case reports in which the patients were diagnosed with ulnar nerve compression at Guyon's canal. During surgical decompression of the canal, the investigators encountered an anomalous transverse muscle located deep to the palmaris brevis muscle. The origin in both cases differed slightly; however, the muscle in both cases inserted into the hypothenar fascia. Release of this muscle resulted in improvement of their symptoms.

The above cases are just a few of the many reported cases of hypothenar muscle anomalies. Understanding these anatomic variations of the hypothenar eminence is important for the surgeon because such structures may confuse the surgeon during wrist or palm procedures. For example, these distinct muscle anomalies may be encountered during a Guyon canal release, extended carpal tunnel release, or palmar fasciectomy.[10] Also, these anomalies should be considered in the differential diagnosis of patients with ulnar nerve entrapment at the level of the wrist because often they are misdiagnosed on magnetic resonance imaging as a ganglion cyst or lipoma.[12]

VASCULAR ANATOMY OF THE HYPOTHENAR MUSCLES

The arterial supply of the hypothenar muscles is provided by the ulnar artery and its branches.[13–15] The ulnar artery divides into superficial and deep branches as it enters the palm. The superficial ulnar branch makes up the superficial palmar arch (SPA), and the deep branch makes up the deep palmar arch (DPA) of the hand.[14]

In the most recent cadaveric study, Murata and colleagues[16] reported on 4 anatomic variations of the ulnar artery at the Guyon canal (Fig. 1).[14,16–24] Their findings are similar to prior studies; however, there is disagreement in the literature regarding the incidence of these variations.[14,17,24] In the most common pattern (type 1, 49%), there is an artery accompanying the deep branch of the ulnar nerve (AADBUN) traveling through the canal. This deep arterial branch continues distally as the DPA. During its course through the canal, the deep branch provides feeder vessels to the ADM, ODM, and FDM. In all the specimens, the superficial branch of the ulnar artery continued into the palm as the SPA distal to the deep branch.[16]

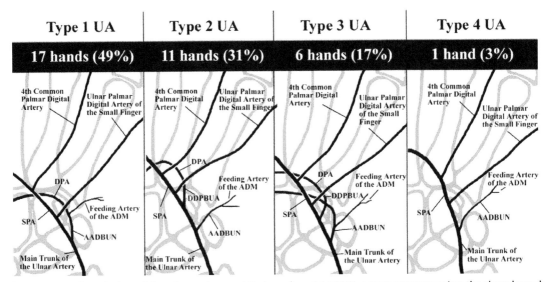

Fig. 1. Anatomic variation of the ulnar artery and its branches. AADBUN, artery accompanying the deep branch of the ulnar nerve; DDPBUA, distal deep palmar branch of the ulnar artery. (*From* Murata K, Tamai M, Gupta A. Anatomic study of arborization patterns of the ulnar artery in Guyon's canal. J Hand Surg Am 2006;31:258–63; with permission.)

In the type 2 pattern (31%), the ulnar artery gave off 2 deep branches. The AADBUN did not form the deep arch of the hand. Instead, the AADBUN became the terminal branch supplying blood to the ADM. In addition, there was a distal deep palmar branch of the ulnar artery (DDPBUA), which entered the midpalmar space between the flexor tendon sheath of the small finger and the FDM. This branch continued distally as the DPA, which provided feeder branches to the ODM. The FDM received its blood supply from a feeder branch off the SPA.[16]

The DDPBUA has been identified in previous studies as well. In one of the largest cadaveric studies of the hand, Coleman and Anson[17] noted a similar inferior deep branch being present in 63% of 200 specimens. König and colleagues[14] reported a second distal branch located deep to the superficial branch, which formed the DPA in 18 of 23 specimens.

In Murata and colleagues' study, type 3 (17%) was not as common. In this pattern, the AADBUN and DDPBUA both form the DPA. The FDM and ADM received their blood supply from the AADBUN in most cases. The artery to the ODM originated from the DDPBUA.[16]

Type 4 was the least common, being present in only 1 specimen (3%). In this pattern, the AADBUN was the feeding vessel to the ADM. In fact, there was no DPA or DDPBUA. The SPA provided the blood supply to the FDM and ODM.[16]

In the findings described above, Murata and colleagues[16] provided a detailed description of

the ulnar artery and its branching patterns within Guyon's canal. Although they pointed out that the use of embalmed specimens was one of the limitations of their study, it remains one of the larger cadaveric studies investigating the ulnar artery in the palm with such meticulous detail.

The differences reported in the branching patterns of the ulnar artery only demonstrate the complexity of the hand's vascularity. No two cadaveric studies are the same; however, similarities of these patterns exist within the literature. It is important for the surgeon to understand that these patterns are present especially when treating disorders of the hypothenar eminence or when using a hypothenar muscle for tendon transfer surgery.

NERVE ANATOMY AND INNERVATION OF THE HYPOTHENAR MUSCLES

The ulnar nerve is responsible for the motor innervation to the hypothenar muscles.[15] The course of the ulnar nerve within the palm is variable. The classic teaching has been that the ulnar nerve divides into the superficial sensory and deep branches proximal to the hiatus of the Guyon canal. The superficial branch then travels over and superficial to the hypothenar muscles where it later branches into the fourth common digital nerve and the ulnar proper digital nerve of the small finger. The deep branch of the ulnar nerve (DBUN) travels through the canal and around the hook of the hamate where it provides motor innervation to the hypothenar muscles. From the cadaveric studies of the recent years, now it is known that there is variability in the path of the ulnar nerve and the arborization pattern of the DBUN.[4]

In a study by Blair and colleagues,[25] 21 cadaveric specimens were dissected to determine the course of the ulnar nerve and the branching pattern of the DBUN within the palm. They noted that the bifurcation of the ulnar nerve occurred near the distal aspect of the Guyon canal at the level of the pisohamate ligament. The deep motor branch follows the medial wall of the hook of hamate and continues distally. In 81% of the specimens, it travels between the FDM and ADM. In 19% of the specimens, the DBUN passes under abductor fibers that originate from the hook of the hamate, and in 1 specimen, the DBUN passed under both the ADM and FDM, which had a common origin.

Once the DBUN passes between the FDM and ADM, it then travels under the medial border of the FDM. When connective tissue bridging the abductor fascia to the flexor fascia was visualized, the DBUN passed underneath the FDM. After it passes under the FDM, the DBUN then enters the ODM. Variations in its path at this point are the following: either it passes between the superficial and deep muscle layers or when bridging fibrous tissue is present, it enters the ODM proximal to these fibrous bands. After innervating the ODM, the DBUN then continues laterally into the deep palmar space.[25]

The branching pattern of the DBUN to the hypothenar muscles demonstrates greater variability than its actual course. The DBUN gives either 1 large main branch or up to 4 small main branches. In 19% of the specimens, the DBUN had 1 main branch to the hypothenar muscles, and in 66% of the specimens, the DBUN supplied 2 main branches to the hypothenar muscle, making this the most common branching pattern observed (**Fig. 2**). Also, there were 2 specimens in which the DBUN supplied 3 main motor branches, and there was 1 specimen that had 4 main motor branches.[25]

In 17 of the specimens, each hypothenar muscle had at least 1 separate motor branch from the DBUN innervating it. The exception to this was when the muscles shared a common origin. In this case, the adjacent muscles receive cross-innervation from the corresponding motor branch.[25]

In another study investigating hypothenar muscle innervation, Murata and colleagues[4] identified 4 different branching patterns of the motor branch to the ADM (**Fig. 3**). In type 1, the motor branch originated from the DBUN distal to the

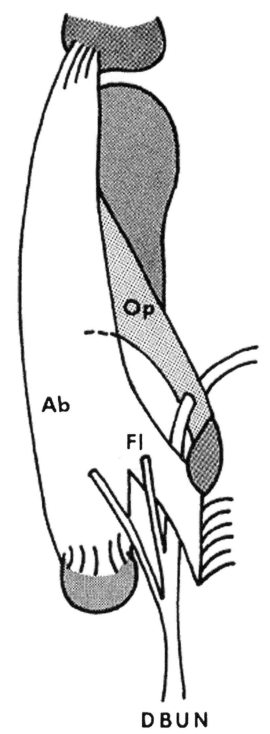

Fig. 2. The most common branching pattern of the DBUN. Of the 2 main motor branches, one terminates in the ADM and the other in the FDM. The DBUN continues into the deep palmar space after supplying motor innervation to the ODM. (*From* Blair WF, Percival KJ, Morecraft R. Distribution pattern of the deep branch of the ulnar nerve in the hypothenar eminence. Clin Orthop 1988;229:294–301; with permission.)

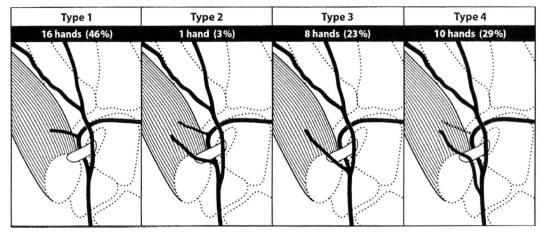

Fig. 3. Branching patterns of motor branch to ADM. (*From* Murata K, Tamai M, Gupta A. Anatomic study of variations of hypothenar muscles and arborization patterns of the ulnar nerve in the hand. J Hand Surg 2004;29: 500–9; with permission.)

canal. This was the most common type. In type 2, there were 2 motor branches with one originating proximal to the canal and the other originating distal to the canal. This was the least common type seen. In type 3, the ulnar nerve trifurcated within the canal into the superficial branch, DBUN, and motor branch to the ADM. In type 4, the motor branch to the ADM originated from the ulnar nerve well proximal to the opening of the Guyon canal.

In addition to the variability of the ulnar nerve distribution to the hypothenar muscles, there has been reported cases in which the median nerve crosses over and provides motor innervation to these muscles as well. The classic description of the Martin-Gruber connection refers to an anomalous motor branch crossover from the median nerve (usually the anterior interosseous nerve) to the ulnar nerve in the proximal forearm.[26,27] Seradge and Seradge[28] described a hypothenar motor branch from the median nerve that was identified within the carpal tunnel. This anomalous motor branch exited through the TCL where it innervated the ADM. The importance of these nerve anomalies is unknown. Being aware of their existence helps explain unusual physical findings unexplained by pathology or normal anatomy.

SUMMARY

Variation in motor nerve distribution of the hypothenar muscles makes surgery to the ulnar side of the palm more challenging. To avoid injury to nerve branches, knowledge of these differences is imperative. In certain procedures, like an opposition transfer of the ADM to the thumb, the motor and

sensory branches of the ulnar nerve should be dissected before mobilization of the muscle and/ or tendon.[4] This careful dissection helps protect the patient from an iatrogenic nerve injury. This is an example in which a basic understanding of these variations is useful during the surgical approach. Perhaps studying the trends of these anatomic differences helps the surgeon with preoperative planning so that he or she will be prepared for any unusual encounters intraoperatively.

REFERENCES

1. Blum AG, Zabel JP, Kohlmann R, et al. Pathologic conditions of the hypothenar eminence: evaluation with multidetector CT and MR imaging. Radiographics 2006;26:1021–44.
2. Pevny T, Rayan GM, Egle D. Ligamentous and tendinous support of the pisiform, anatomic and biomechanical study. J Hand Surg Am 1995;20:299–304.
3. Rotman MB, Donovan JP. Practical anatomy of the carpal tunnel. Hand Clin 2002;18:219–30.
4. Murata K, Tamai M, Gupta A. Anatomic study of variations of hypothenar muscles and arborization patterns of the ulnar nerve in the hand. J Hand Surg 2004;29:500–9.
5. Kung J, Budoff JE, Wei ML, et al. The origins of the thenar and hypothenar muscles. J Hand Surg Br 2005;30:475.
6. Gartsman GM, Kovach JC, Crouch CC, et al. Carpal arch alteration after carpal tunnel release. J Hand Surg Am 1986;11:372–4.
7. Netscher D, Steadman AK, Thornby J, et al. Temporal changes in grip and pinch strength after open carpal tunnel release and the effect of ligament reconstruction. J Hand Surg Am 1998;23:48–54.

8. Brand PW, Hollister AM. Clinical mechanics of the hand. 3rd edition. St Louis (MO): Mosby Inc; 1999. p. 173–5.
9. Fahrer M. Anatomy of the karate chop. Bull Hosp Jt Dis Orthop Inst 1984;44:189–98.
10. Curry B, Kuz J. A new variation of abductor digiti minimi accessorius. J Hand Surg Am 2000;25:585–7.
11. Failla JM. The hypothenar abductor muscle: an anomalous intrinsic muscle compressing the ulnar nerve. J Hand Surg Am 1996;21:366–8.
12. Turner MS, Caird DM. Anomalous muscle and ulnar nerve compression at the wrist. Hand 1977;9:140–2.
13. Guyon F. Note sur une disposition anatomique proper a la face anterieure de la region du poignet et non encore decrite. Bull MCm Sot Anat 1861;6: 184–6 [in French].
14. König PS, Hage JJ, Bloem JJ, et al. Variations of the ulnar nerve and ulnar artery in Guyon's canal: a cadaveric study. J Hand Surg Am 1994;19:617–22.
15. Kaplan EB. Functional and surgical anatomy of the hand. Philadelphia: Lippincott; 1953. p. 74–6.
16. Murata K, Tamai M, Gupta A. Anatomic study of arborization patterns of the ulnar artery in Guyon's canal. J Hand Surg Am 2006;31:258–63.
17. Coleman SS, Anson BJ. Arterial patterns in the hand based upon a study of 650 specimens. Surg Gynecol Obstet 1961;113:409–24.
18. Denman EE. The anatomy of the space of Guyon. Hand 1978;10:69–76.
19. Karlsson S, Niechajev IA. Arterial anatomy of the upper extremity. Acta Radiol Diagn 1982;23:115–21.
20. Gelberman RH, Panagis JS, Taleisnik J, et al. The arterial anatomy of the human carpus. Part I: the extraosseous vascularity. J Hand Surg Am 1983;8: 367–75.
21. Gross MS, Gelberman RH. The anatomy of the distal ulnar tunnel. Clin Orthop 1985;196:238–47.
22. Zeiss J, Jakab E, Khimji T, et al. The ulnar tunnel at the wrist (Guyon's canal): normal MR anatomy and variants. AJR Am J Roentgenol 1992;158:1081–5.
23. Lindsey JT, Watumull D. Anatomic study of the ulnar nerve and related vascular anatomy at Guyon's canal: a practical classification system. J Hand Surg Am 1996;21:626–33.
24. Gellman H, Bott MJ, Shankwiler J, et al. Arterial patterns of the deep and superficial palmar arches. Clin Orthop 2001;383:41–6.
25. Blair WF, Percival KJ, Morecraft R. Distribution pattern of the deep branch of the ulnar nerve in the hypothenar eminence. Clin Orthop 1988;229: 294–301.
26. Gruber W. Ueber die Verbindung Des Nervns Medianus met dem nervus ulnaris am unterarme des menschen und der sangethiete. Arch Anat Phisiol Wiss Med 1870;37:501 [in German].
27. Martin R. Tal om Nervus allmanna egenskaper i Mannsikans Kropp. Stockholm (Sweden): Lars Salvius; 1763.
28. Seradge H, Seradge E. Median innervated hypothenar muscle: anomalous branch of median nerve in the carpal tunnel. J Hand Surg Am 1990;15: 356–9.

Restoration of Opposition

Martin A. Posner, MD[a],*, Deepak Kapila, MD[b]

KEYWORDS

- Opposition • Thenar muscles • Intrinsic muscles
- Opposition tendon transfers

Opposition of the thumb has been referred to as "the most important component of normal thumb function."[1] Stirling Bunnell[2] defined it as "when the thumb is diametrically opposite to the fingers with the thumb pulp facing fingers and the thumb nail is parallel to the volar surfaces of the fingers." Opposition is at its maximum when the distal pulp of the thumb is directly opposite the distal pulp of the middle finger, regardless of the distance between the 2 digits. It is therefore the same when the thumb and middle finger are grasping a marble or a baseball. Although grasp between the thumb and ring and little fingers is a common hand function, the middle finger is the reference point for opposition. With opposition to the ring and little fingers, the fingers are moving toward the thumb rather than the reverse; the thumb does not move into greater opposition when it approaches those fingers.

MECHANICS OF OPPOSITION

Opposition begins with the thumb in its resting position, a position of 90° pronation to the plane of the fingers. Therefore, for the thumb to achieve maximum opposition, an additional pronation of 90° is required that occurs in a curvilinear manner and encompasses 3 motions: abduction, flexion, and pronation. Abduction occurs primarily at the trapeziometacarpal (TM) joint and is the angle between the first and second metacarpals in the sagittal plane. At its maximum, the angle approximates 40° to 50°. The contribution of the metacarpophalangeal (MP) joint, a condyloid joint, depends on the degree of normal ligament laxity

and the morphology of the joint, especially the head of the metacarpal. The MP joints in fingers are also condyloid joints, but the curvature of the metacarpal heads is significantly greater than the MP joints of thumbs. Finger MP joints are therefore capable of a wide arc of abduction/adduction. The metacarpal heads in thumb MP joints are usually flat, which limits abduction/adduction; abduction ranges from a few degrees to 20° to 25°. The interphalangeal (IP) joint, a ginglymus or hinge joint, contributes nothing. Total abduction of the thumb is therefore variable and can range from 40° to 50°, provided by the TM joint, to 70° to 75°, when there is also a contribution from the MP joint.

The muscles involved in thumb abduction, the first component of opposition, are essentially the intrinsic muscles in the thenar eminence: the abductor pollicis brevis (APB), the superficial or radial head of the flexor pollicis brevis (FPB), and the opponens pollicis. The only thenar muscle not involved in abduction is the deep or ulnar head of the FPB. The extrinsic abductor pollicis longus (APL), despite its name, contributes little. APL's primary function is extension of the thumb ray (in the coronal plane) via its insertion into the base of the first metacarpal. Its contribution to thumb abduction is when a tendon slip(s) inserts volar to the TM joint; this rarely occurs. Rather than abducting the thumb, the APL extends the first metacarpal, which is important for maintaining the longitudinal arch of the thumb. Without that arch, the MP joint usually becomes secondarily hyperextended and the IP joint goes into a flexed position, resulting in a zigzag deformity. This is commonly seen in the patient with TM joint arthritis whose

[a] Division of Hand Surgery, New York University–Hospital for Joint Diseases, 301 East 17 Street, New York, NY 10003, USA
[b] 7050 Northwest 4 Street, Plantation, FL 33317, USA
* Corresponding author.
E-mail address: martin.posner@nyumc.org

Hand Clin 28 (2012) 27–44
doi:10.1016/j.hcl.2011.09.004
0749-0712/12/$ – see front matter © 2012 Elsevier Inc. All rights reserved.

APL tendon becomes attenuated by the inflammation and the joint is radially subluxated. The APL is therefore misnamed. A more appropriate name would be the *extensor metacarpus primus*, the extensor of the first metacarpal.

The flexion component of opposition involves all 3 thumb joints. TM joint flexion permits positioning of the head of the thumb metacarpal in the same sagittal plane as the head of the middle finger metacarpal, MP joint flexion facilitates grasping objects of different sizes with less flexion obviously required for large objects than for small objects, and IP joint flexion depends on the prehensile activity being performed. For pulp-to-pulp pinch, the IP joint is extended or is in slight flexion, and for tip-to-tip pinch, it is in greater flexion. The muscles that contribute to the flexion component of opposition are the intrinsic thumb muscles with the exception of the opponens pollicis, which inserts entirely on the first metacarpal. For forceful flexion, there are important contributions from the adductor pollicis, an intrinsic thumb muscle that is not in the thenar eminence and is innervated by the ulnar nerve, and from the extrinsic flexor pollicis longus (FPL).

The third component of opposition, pronation, occurs around a longitudinal axis through the center of the TM joint. Pronation essentially occurs simultaneously with flexion and abduction of the TM joint caused by the configurations of its articular surfaces and ligaments. The TM joint is a concavoconvex joint that is commonly referred to as a saddle joint. Based on its anatomic configuration, a saddle joint permits motions in 2 planes: flexion/extension and abduction/adduction. The motions can be compared with a cowboy sitting snugly in a Western saddle who is able to bend forward and backward and shift side to side but is unable to turn because of the high cantle of the saddle in the rear and the prominent horn in the front. For him to turn or rotate, the cowboy must first lift himself from the saddle seat by pushing down against the stirrups. It is much easier for a rider to turn in an English saddle, which has a lower cantle and no horn. The articular surfaces of a human saddle joint (TM joint) are shallow and therefore more closely resemble an English saddle than a Western saddle. It is the shallow articular configurations and the anatomy of the ligaments that provide sufficient laxity to the TM joint to permit rotation, often referred to as circumduction, the third component of opposition.

For opposition (a combination of abduction, flexion, and pronation) to be effective, the thenar intrinsic muscles, including the APB, radial head of the FPB, and opponens pollicis, must function. The APB is the most important muscle for opposition. It abducts, flexes, and rotates the metacarpal; abducts and flexes the proximal phalanx; and extends the IP joint. The radial head of the FPB is a weak abductor that is not nearly as effective as the APB, and the opponens pollicis is even less effective. The opponens pollicis abducts, flexes, and rotates the metacarpal similar to the APB but has no effect distal to the MP joint because its insertion is solely on the first metacarpal. The opponens pollicis is the least important intrinsic muscle for thumb opposition, and is the reason why Emanuel Kaplan, the great anatomist and first Chief of the Division of Hand Surgery at New York University Hospital for Joint Diseases, objected to the term "opponensplasty". Kaplan taught that when surgery was performed for absence of thenar muscle function, the objective was to restore opposition and not restore function of the opponens pollicis; He often stated, "Why name an operation for the least important thenar muscle?" He preferred the term "opposition tendon transfer" because it accurately described the objective of the procedure; it is the term used by Kaplan's students and the one taught to residents and fellows.

GENERAL PRINCIPLES OF OPPOSITION

Hand function essentially involves the ability to grasp (grip and prehension are synonymous terms) objects that vary in size and weight. There are 2 types of grasp, power grasp and precision grasp, and the thumb has an important role in both. In power grasp, the thumb is in an adducted position and often provides a stabilizing force as when using a hammer; the fingers impart most of the grasp force to the handle. In precision grasp, often referred to as pinch, the thumb tip contacts the tip of 1 or more fingers. For 2-point pinch, it is the tip of the index finger, and, for 3-point or chuck pinch, it is the tips of the index and middle fingers. Key pinch, when the pulp of the distal segment of the thumb is pressed firmly against the side of the proximal segment of the index finger, is a form of power grasp.

Opposition is not grasp but a preparatory position to grasp that requires the thenar intrinsic muscles (with the exception of the ulnar head of the FPB) to place the thumb in that position. From that preparatory position, the thumb can participate in power and precision grip activities. Thumb opposition and grasp are therefore 2 separate stages. When both are compromised and reconstructive surgery is necessary, restoring opposition is the first priority. Opposition does not require a strong tendon transfer. Any tendon capable of moving a passively mobile thumb has sufficient force to be an effective opposition tendon transfer. Only when the force of grasp is impaired is a strong tendon transfer required.[3] Power grasp, and that includes key pinch, is rarely significantly compromised in a low median nerve injury because the functions of the adductor pollicis innervated by the ulnar nerve and FPL innervated by the median nerve in the proximal forearm are not impaired. If the staging of the reconstructive procedures for a low median nerve injury was reversed and a strong tendon transfer was first used for opposition, there would be a risk of causing a flexion deformity of the TM and/or MP joint.[3] Restoration of pinch is discussed in Chapter 6.

PREOPERATIVE ASSESSMENT

Selecting the optimum treatment for the patient with paralysis of the thenar intrinsic muscles depends on a variety of factors that include the cause of the paralysis, the duration and severity of the functional impairment, and any other significant medical problems. Congenital aplasia or hypoplasia of the thenar muscles is obviously a very different problem than paralysis of those muscles following a median nerve laceration when there are also profound sensory deficits on the tactile surfaces of the thumb, index finger, and middle finger. When intrinsic muscle paralysis is the result of a nerve laceration, a neurorrhaphy is preferable to a tendon transfer, provided that the procedure is performed within a time frame that permits muscle reinnervation. Motor end plates of denervated muscles undergo fibrosis at approximately 18 months. Therefore, regenerating motor axons must reach those end plates before that time. A median nerve repair at the wrist has a better prognosis for reinnervating paralyzed intrinsic muscles than a similar injury in the elbow or in the proximal forearm because the regenerating axons have a shorter distance to travel. Using the generally accepted guide that regenerating motor axons progress at the rate of 1 mm a day or 25 mm (1 inch) a month, a reasonable estimate can be made for the time that muscle reinnervation can be expected and if it will be within the 18-month time frame. For chronic injuries, the time that has lapsed from the date of the original injury is added to the distance the regenerating axons must travel when deciding if a neurorrhaphy would be the appropriate treatment option. It would be the appropriate option for a nerve injury at the wrist that is 6 months old, but it would not be appropriate for an injury that is 18 months old, because by the time the regenerating motor axons reached the intrinsic muscles, the end plates would likely be fibrotic. The prognosis for muscle reinnervation is also dependent on the type of injury. A neurorrhaphy for a sharp lacerating injury generally has a better prognosis than for a ripping injury caused by a power saw or for a high-velocity injury, such as a gunshot wound, because both types of injuries result in large zones of nerve damage, and repair usually requires an interposition nerve graft.

The extent of the functional deficit in the patient with thenar muscle paralysis must be carefully evaluated before deciding on a course of treatment or whether any treatment is needed. Frequently, when the paralysis is secondary to a median nerve injury, the sensory deficit is far more disabling than the motor deficit. This is especially true in those patients who can still abduct their thumbs through the action of the radial head of the FPB, which frequently has a dual innervation from both median and ulnar nerves.[4] Although these patients are unable to position their thumbs in complete opposition, the abduction component of opposition is usually sufficient and there is no need for an opposition tendon transfer. However, when there is significant functional impairment and an opposition tendon transfer is warranted, it is important to evaluate the activities of that particular patient to determine the optimum type of transfer.

Before any tendon transfer, preoperative passive mobility of the thumb should be complete or almost complete; passive abduction is more important than passive rotation. An adduction contracture of the first web space must first be corrected and this can often be accomplished with nonoperative measures that involve passive abduction thumb exercises. To be effective, the patient should do the exercises frequently for brief periods, generally 10 repetitions every hour or even every half hour during the day. It is also important that the exercises are performed properly with the patient applying an abduction force to the ulnar side of the head of the metacarpal and not to the ulnar side of the proximal phalanx, which can result in stretching of the ulnar collateral ligament of the MP joint and lead to instability. Supervised therapy with a hand therapist is usually beneficial. Those treatments are an adjunct and not a substitute for the patient's own exercises. A static C-shaped splint for the thumb web space is used when the patient is not exercising. A dynamic abduction splint is also effective and is generally worn for 20 to 30 minutes several times during the day. As with passive abduction exercises, the forces applied by static and dynamic abduction splints must be against the ulnar side of the metacarpal head and not against the ulnar side of the phalanx to avoid causing instability of the MP joint. When nonoperative measures are unsuccessful, surgery is necessary and precedes the tendon transfer. The surgical treatment of adduction contractures is discussed in Chapter 8.

HISTORY OF OPPOSITION TENDON TRANSFERS

The history of tendon transfers for thumb opposition dates back to the early part of the twentieth century when in 1918 Steindler[5] split the FPL, leaving the ulnar half of the tendon insertion intact and rerouting the radial half of the tendon through a hole in the flexor tendon sheath and inserting it on the radial side of the proximal phalanx. The transfer was not effective because one muscle cannot perform such different functions as thumb flexion and thumb opposition. During the 1920s to 1940s, various other tendon transfers were recommended and many used a flexor digitorum superficialis (FDS) as the motor. In 1922, Krukenberg[6] split the FDS to a middle finger, left the insertion of the ulnar half of the tendon intact, and transferred the radial half of the tendon to the thumb metacarpal. As with Steindler's procedure, the transfer was not effective in improving thumb opposition.

Over the ensuing years, contributions to restoring thenar muscle function were made by other surgeons, and 3 deserve special recognition: Royle, Bunnell, and Thompson.[3] In 1938, Royle[7] recognized the importance of transferring an entire FDS tendon rather than just half the tendon, which had been recommended earlier and was not effective, because the half that was left intact at its insertion into the middle phalanx interfered with the function of the other half that was transferred to the thumb. Royle's concept of using 1 FDS tendon to do 1 function was correct, but the direction of the transfer was not effective to restore opposition. Similar to what Steindler had recommended, Royle simply transferred the tendon through a hole in the tendon sheath of the thumb and attached it to the radial side of the proximal phalanx of the thumb. The transfer produced little thumb abduction and no pronation.

Bunnell[2] also used an FDS as a motor and modified his surgical technique several times before he published his classic article on the subject in 1938. Bunnell recognized the important role of the APB in thumb opposition and that the direction of its muscle fibers was toward the pisiform bone. To replicate this line of pull, Bunnell rerouted the FDS through a pulley constructed in the flexor carpi ulnaris (FCU) tendon near its insertion into the pisiform, and, to maximize thumb pronation, he inserted the FDS tendon into the ulnar base of the proximal phalanx.

In 1942, Thompson[8] modified Royle's earlier procedure by also improving the direction of the transfer. He rerouted the FDS at the distal end of the transverse carpal ligament and at the ulnar border of the palmar fascia and then transferred it subcutaneously across the palm to the thumb MP joint where he split it into 2 slips. One slip was inserted into the hood mechanism over the proximal phalanx and the other slip into a drill hole in the neck of the metacarpal. Because Thompson's procedure was a modification of Royle's procedure, it is commonly referred to as the Royle-Thompson procedure. A major difference between the Bunnell and Royle-Thompson procedures is the line of pull of the tendon transfers. In the Bunnell procedure, the line of pull is toward the pisiform along the course of the APB, the key muscle for opposition, whereas in the Royle-Thompson procedure, the pull is more distal along the radial head of the FPB, which provides greater flexion and adduction to the thumb but less abduction.

Opposition tendon transfers using motors other than the FDS have been recommended, and one of the earliest was transfer of the abductor digiti quinti (ADQ), which is also referred to as the abductor digiti minimi (ADM), an intrinsic muscle innervated by the ulnar nerve in the hypothenar area of the palm. Huber proposed the procedure in 1921 and Nicolaysen just 1 year later in 1922.[9,10] Transfers using other tendons have been recommended, as well as different methods of attachments. The chronology of the most significant procedures is as follows:

1921, Steindler[5]: radial half of FPL through tendon sheath to radial side of phalanx

1921, Ney[11]: palmaris longus (PL) or flexor carpi radialis (FCR) attached to extensor pollicis brevis (EPB), which is transposed into carpal tunnel

1921, Taylor[12]: extensor digiti quinti proprius (EDQP) around ulnar border of hand to radial side of thumb metacarpal

1921, Huber[9]; 1922, Nicolaysen[10]: ADQ in hypothenar eminence to APB

1922, Krukenberg[6]: radial half of FDS (middle) rerouted as described by Steindler

1924, Lyle[13]: FCR to EPB and radial half of FPL to radial side of proximal phalanx

1926, Howell[14]: FPL transected at wrist, rerouted around the ulna to radial side of the thumb

1929, Camitz[15]: PL + palmar aponeurosis to radial side of thumb MP joint

1937, Royle[7]: FDS (ring) through tendon sheath to radial side of proximal phalanx

1938, Bunnell[2]: FDS (ring) through pulley in FCU to ulnar base of proximal phalanx

1942, Thompson[8]: FDS (ring) rerouted ulnar border of palmar aponeurosis to the thumb

1947, Phalen and Miller[16]: extensor carpi ulnaris (ECU) to rerouted EPB

1956, Zancolli[17]: extensor pollicis longus (EPL) through carpal tunnel into APB

1959, Riordan[18]: insertion of FDS; one-half into APB and the other half into EPL

1962, Henderson[19]: ECU, extensor carpi radialis longus (ECRL), extensor carpi radialis brevis (ECRB), or brachioradialis (BR) prolonged with a graft or to EPB

1967, Makin[20]: translocation of intact FPL through an osteotomy in the proximal phalanx

1968, Tubiana and Valentin[21]: EPL around FCR superficial to carpal tunnel into APB

1969, Schneider[22]: described transfer of EDQP proposed by Taylor in 1921

1973, Mangus[23]: FPL around FCU to APB, tenodesis of FPL at IP joint

1973, Burkhalter[24]: extensor indicis proprius (EIP) around ulnar border of hand to APB

Most of these procedures are primarily of historical interest. Those transfers that are currently relevant and are most frequently performed are discussed.

OPPOSITION TENDON TRANSFERS
Flexor Digitorum Superficialis Transfers

The Thompson-Royle procedure is still used for certain clinical problems, especially after combined injuries to median and ulnar nerves when there is paralysis of all the intrinsic thumb muscles, commonly referred to as the intrinsic minus thumb. The FDS tendon to the ring finger is identified through an incision at the base of the finger as well as more proximally through a 3-cm longitudinal incision along the radial border of the hypothenar eminence where it emerges from the carpal tunnel. The tendon is transected through the distal incision, withdrawn through the proximal incision, brought superficial to the ulnar side of the palmar

fascia, and then passed subcutaneously across the palm to the thumb. In the original procedure, the FDS insertion was split, and, as previously discussed, one slip was inserted into the extensor hood over the proximal phalanx and the other slip into the metacarpal.

The route of the transfer is essentially transverse across the palm, and the FDS roughly parallels the path of the muscle fibers in the superficial head of the FPB. The transfer, therefore, more effectively flexes the thumb than abducts it. It also stabilizes the MP joint, and it is for this reason that the procedure is used for combined median and ulnar nerve palsies. However, the Royle-Thompson procedure is not as effective as a transfer performed solely to improve thumb opposition or to improve thumb adduction. When restoration of both functions is necessary, it is often preferable to perform a separate tendon transfer for each.

The Bunnell opposition transfer is a commonly performed transfer because it effectively restores thumb opposition (**Fig. 1**). As previously noted, its line of pull parallels the fibers of the APB toward the pisiform. This is accomplished by redirecting the FDS tendon through a pulley constructed in the FCU tendon near its insertion into the pisiform. The FDS is harvested through a transverse incision in the distal palm, midway between the distal palmar crease and the flexion crease at the base of the ring finger. In some cases, the FDS tendon in the middle finger is used and then the incision is made at the base of that finger. Two additional incisions are required, one on the volar aspect of the distal forearm and wrist and the other over the dorsum of the MP joint of the thumb. It is preferable to prepare both operative sites, including the subcutaneous tunnel between them, which is made with a curved mosquito and/or curved hemostat clamp, before the FDS tendon is harvested to minimize the time that it is left exposed.

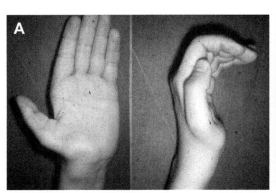
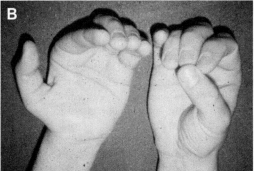

Fig. 1. Congenital absence of the thenar muscles in the left hand of a 25-year-old recent immigrant to the United States who never had treatment in his native country. (*A*) Complete flattening of the thenar eminence with no active thumb abduction. (*B*) Comparative photo with the right hand shows normal opposition of that thumb.

Through the incision in the palm, the proximal pulley of the flexor tendon sheath is identified, and the FDS is isolated from the flexor digitorum profundus (FDP). With the donor finger in maximum flexion at the proximal IP (PIP) joint, traction is placed on the FDS, and it is transected as far distally as possible to leave a distal remnant of the tendon of 2 to 3 cm. Transecting the FDS in this manner is preferable to detaching it at its insertion, which destroys the vincula and can compromise the blood supply to the overlying FDP tendon.[25] It can also lead to a hyperextension or swan-neck deformity of the PIP joint. Swan-neck deformities are much more likely to occur in individuals with supple joints that can easily be passively hyperextended than in individuals whose hands are thick and brawny and whose fingers are stiffer. Even in the patient with supple joints, cutting the FDS in the method described leaves a distal remnant of tendon that usually scars to the tendon sheath and results in a slight tenodesis of the PIP joint that rarely exceeds 10° to 15° and is not a functional impairment. More severe flexion contractures are prevented by simply passively extending the PIP joint on the first postoperative day and encouraging the patient to actively and passively exercise while the splint is in place.

The FDS is withdrawn through the incision in the palm and then through the incision in the forearm where the pulley in the FCU is constructed. The distal 4 to 5 cm of the FCU tendon is split longitudinally with a #11 scalpel blade, and the radial half of the split tendon is cut proximally. This portion of the tendon is looped and passed through a slit in the intact distal portion of the FCU to which it is sutured. To avoid making the loop too large, which would permit the FDS tendon to shift away from the pisiform, or too small, which can interfere with its gliding, the FDS tendon is passed through the loop before the loop is sutured to the intact portion of the FCU. However, before doing so, the FDS tendon is passed around the intact portion of the FCU. Rerouting the FDS first around the FCU and then through the pulley is an important technical component of the operation (Fig. 2). One without the other can compromise the result. Rerouting the FDS around the intact portion of the FCU ensures that it remains on the ulnar side of the wrist and cannot shift radially, and passing it through a pulley close to the pisiform ensures that its direction of pull is in line with the muscle fibers of the APB and does not pull more proximally, which would compromise thumb pronation. If the carpal tunnel is decompressed at the time of the tendon transfer, the palmar fascia is sutured before the FDS tendon is passed subcutaneously across the palm.

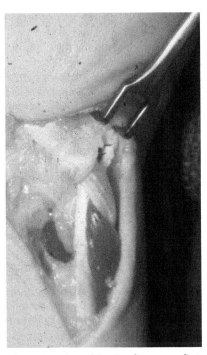

Fig. 2. The FDS tendon of the ring finger was first passed around the ulnar border of the FCU and then through a pulley constructed in the distal portion of that tendon.

There are a variety of methods of attaching the FDS to the thumb; they can be divided into single- and dual-insertion techniques.[26] Single-insertion techniques are the most frequently performed and are commonly used for isolated median nerve palsies. Bunnell recommended that the tendon be inserted into the ulnar side of the base of the proximal phalanx as a means to achieve not only maximum abduction but also maximum pronation. The transfer should pass directly over the dorsum of the MP joint and not distal to the joint. The authors usually prefer this technique (Fig. 3). Inserting the tendon into bone requires more careful tensioning than attaching it to soft tissues because it is more difficult to correct if the tension is incorrect. When an FDS transfer is inserted into the proximal phalanx and is too loose, the tendon is simply shortened and reinserted, but a transfer that is too tight may require using a different FDS because the tendon is now too short. Biomechanical studies have shown that the TM joint passively pronates when the thumb is actively abducted and flexed, and opposition is thought to be as effective when the transfer is attached to the APB insertion on the radial side of the MP joint as when it is inserted into the ulnar base of the proximal phalanx.[27] The APB tendon is the most common site of insertion for a variety of opposition transfers for isolated median nerve palsies.[28–30] A dual insertion into the APB tendon and into the thumb

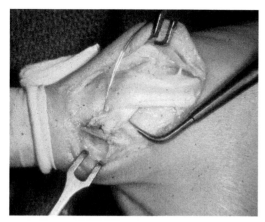

Fig. 3. The FDS tendon was passed under the extensor tendons on the dorsum of the thumb and sutured into the ulnar base of the proximal phalanx with the wrist in slight flexion and the thumb in maximum opposition.

extensor mechanism is sometimes necessary when extension of the MP and IP joints must be improved in addition to opposition.[31]

Regardless of the method of insertion, tension of the transfer is adjusted with the wrist in neutral or approximately 30° flexion and the thumb in opposition to the middle finger. Gauging the correct amount of tension is as much the art of hand surgery as it is a science. An effective method is to exert maximum traction on the tendon end that is held in a clamp, measure the distance that the tendon moved distally, and then attach the tendon with sufficient traction on it to equal about half that distance. Tension is correct when with passive wrist extension the thumb moves into complete opposition. If passive wrist extension is restricted, the transfer is too tight and it should be resutured in a more lengthened position. As previously noted, this is more difficult when the transfer is sutured into the proximal phalanx because there may be insufficient tendon remaining to resuture it in a lengthened position. If, however, thumb abduction is less with passive wrist extension than can be achieved by passively abducting the thumb, the transfer should be shortened. Thumb position is also evaluated by moving the wrist into full flexion. If the thumb does not fully adduct, the transfer is too tight and it should be lengthened. It is also important to evaluate the position of the MP joint of the thumb. If the joint flexes more than 25° to 30° with wrist extension, the tendon attachment should be more dorsal, and, if the joint hyperextends with wrist extension, it should be sutured more volar. There are occasional situations when the MP joint is unstable and the tendon transfer snaps it into flexion, hyperextension, or sometimes both. The options in such cases are either to arthrodese the MP joint or to suture the transfer to the radial collateral ligament of the joint. Postoperatively, the wrist is immobilized in 30° to 40° flexion and the thumb in full opposition for 4 weeks. At the end of that period, the splint is removed several times daily for active range of motion exercises and is worn at all other times for an additional 1 to 2 weeks. A C-splint can be used for protection for several more weeks.

The results of a Bunnell opposition transfer are generally excellent in the patient with a low median nerve paralysis whose flexor tendons are intact and who has minimal scarring on the volar aspect of the distal forearm and wrist (**Fig. 4**). There are several

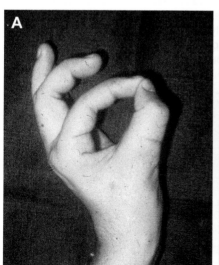
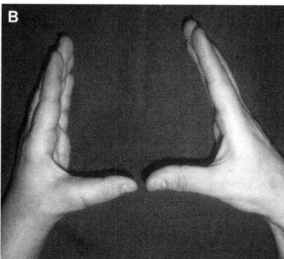

Fig. 4. Postoperative results. (*A*) Complete opposition restored. (*B*) Comparative photo with the right hand showing equal pronation of both thumbs.

disadvantages to the transfer. It is unavailable in the high median nerve injury that results in paralysis of all the FDS muscles, as well as in the high ulnar nerve injury that results in paralysis of the FDP muscles to the ring and little fingers. In the latter situation, the FDS is the only functioning flexor tendon in the ring finger and obviously must be retained. However, the FDS tendon to the middle finger can be substituted because the FDP to that finger is innervated by the median nerve. Another disadvantage of using the ring finger FDS for transfer is a decrease in postoperative power grip. The ring and little fingers are necessary for power grip, whereas the index and middle fingers are more involved with precision grip. If a postoperative decrease in power grip would be detrimental to the patient's hand function, the middle finger FDS should be used instead.[26] Generally, the impact on grip strength is mild regardless of the FDS tendon that is used for the transfer. A potentially more serious functional deficit may occur in those individuals whose activities require independent FDS function, such as some musicians, especially harpists.

A potential technical complication of the procedure is scarring and adherence of the FDS tendon as it passes through the pulley. This complication can be avoided by suturing the loop of the FCU into the intact portion of the tendon with its paratenon surface and not its cut surface in contact with the transfer. Potential complications related to sectioning the donor FDS tendon that can lead to a swan-neck deformity or flexion contracture of the PIP joint were discussed previously.

Extensor Indicis Proprius Transfer

In the patient with total intrinsic muscle paralysis due to combined low median and ulnar nerve injuries, the EIP is often the procedure of choice to restore thumb opposition (**Fig. 5**). The FDS tendons are reserved to correct clawing of the fingers.[3,29,32] The route of an EIP transfer is more direct than that of an FDS transfer for which the path takes a more acute angle as it passes through the pulley in the FCU.[33] By having a more direct line of pull, significantly less force is required for an EIP opposition transfer than for an FDS opposition transfer (approximately 40% less force).[34] Although this is a large percentage, it is not as significant as for a transfer performed to restore the force of grasp. As previously discussed, opposition is not grasp but is a preparatory position to grasp and requires only a force that is sufficient to move a passively mobile thumb.

The EIP tendon is harvested at its insertion through a small transverse incision over the

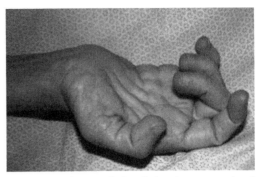

Fig. 5. Postpolio paralysis of the thenar muscles in a 25-year-old woman; finger flexors were weak, and FDS tendons were not suitable for transfer.

dorsum of the index MP joint. The tendon lies to the ulnar side of the extensor digitorum communis (EDC). Some recommend that the EIP should be harvested with a contiguous strip of the extensor hood to ensure that it is of sufficient length to reach its insertion.[24,34] This procedure is usually unnecessary and can cause a problem if the extensor hood is not properly repaired. The EDC could shift radially and result in an extension lag.[26,35] The EIP is usually transected just proximal to the extensor hood, and the distal short stump of the EIP is sutured to the EDC to preserve a balanced extensor pull on the proximal phalanx.[3] Several other incisions are necessary and, as when performing an FDS transfer, it is preferable to make those incisions and prepare the subcutaneous tunnels for passage of the EIP before the tendon is harvested. A second incision approximately 4 cm in length is made over the dorsoulnar side of the forearm, 6 to 10 cm proximal to the ulnar styloid, to visualize the musculotendinous junction of the EIP. The underlying fascia is divided longitudinally, and the EIP tendon is withdrawn (**Fig. 6**). It is important that its muscle belly is freed from the surrounding soft tissues before the tendon is

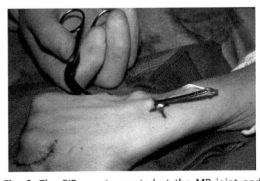

Fig. 6. The EIP was transected at the MP joint and withdrawn through an incision proximal to the extensor retinaculum.

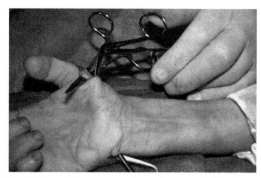

Fig. 7. The EIP was routed to the ulnar side of the wrist and then across the palm and attached to the tendon of the APB.

passed subcutaneously to the third operative site, which is just proximal to the pisiform. Care must be taken to ensure that the EIP muscle is not angulated by any fascial bands in the forearm. A small transverse incision just proximal to the pisiform permits retrieval of the EIP tendon, which is then passed subcutaneously to its site of attachment at the thumb MP joint. Again, care must be taken to ensure that the tendon's path across the palm is in a straight line and that it glides freely. The EIP is then sutured to the APB tendon (**Fig. 7**). Tensioning of the transfer and the postoperative care are the same as for an FDS transfer.

The advantages of an EIP transfer are that there is no loss of grip force because an extensor tendon is used, the FDS tendons are preserved to restore intrinsic muscle function in the fingers if necessary,

and a pulley is not required. The main disadvantage of the procedure is that the patient may lose some independent extension of the index MP joint. This is more theoretical than actual because the remaining EDC tendon usually functions as an independent extensor tendon because it has no junctura tendinum (or a rudimentary junctura tendinum) to the EDC to the adjacent middle finger that can tether it. In most cases, complete and independent MP extension is maintained postoperatively. Even when there is an extension lag, it is rarely more than 20°, which has no functional significance. Another possible disadvantage of the transfer is a technical one. The EIP is usually of sufficient length to reach the insertion site, but there is little extra tendon to spare. Occasionally, it is too short and has to be prolonged with a tendon graft.

Abductor Digiti Quinti Transfer

The ADQ transfer, which is also referred to as the ADM transfer, was first reported by Huber[9] in 1921 and 1 year later in 1922 by Nicolaysen.[10] In terms of longevity, ADQ transfer is the oldest performed opposition tendon transfer. The technical details of the procedure were established by Littler and Cooley in 1963.[30] Although the ADQ is in the hypothenar eminence, is innervated by the ulnar nerve, and abducts the little finger, it has a remarkable similarity to the APB. Because the mass and excursions of both muscles are similar, the ADQ can be used as a substitute for the APB.[36] The primary indication for the procedure is congenital absence of the thenar muscles because, in

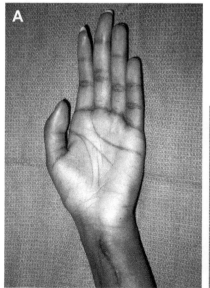

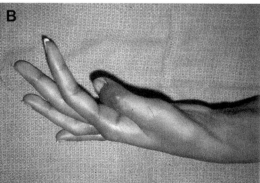

Fig. 8. A 35-year-old woman sustained lacerations of the median nerve and flexor tendons in the distal forearm, which were repaired. (*A*) Protective sensibility restored and good finger flexion. (*B*) No thumb abduction.

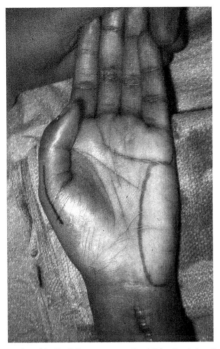

Fig. 9. The skin incisions are marked. The incision in the palm begins on the ulnar side of the little finger and is continued along the entire radial border of the hypothenar eminence into the wrist flexion crease.

scarring about the wrist that is likely to interfere with gliding of tendon transfers, in cases of combined median and radial nerve paralysis, in patients with absence of multiple fingers because of injury or aplasia, and as a means to supplement opposition in a previously pollicized index finger.[3]

The primary operative approach is to expose the entire length of the ADQ in the hypothenar eminence. This is accomplished by an incision made along the ulnar side of the proximal segment of the little finger that is curved radially into the distal palmar crease and is then continued proximally along the entire radial border of the hypothenar eminence to the wrist flexion crease (**Figs. 8** and **9**). The incision is curved ulnarly into the crease for 1 to 2 cm and is then curved proximally and continued over the FCU tendon for an additional 1 to 2 cm. The distal insertions of the ADQ into the proximal phalanx and lateral band of the extensor mechanism are identified and released. The muscle belly of the ADQ is freed distally to proximally, separating it from the underlying flexor digiti quinti. At the proximal end of the ADQ, the neurovascular bundle that enters the muscle on its deep or dorsal surface just distal to the pisiform is identified and protected. A second midaxial incision is made on the radial side of the thumb MP and the tendon of the APB is identified; its muscle is usually pale because of being denervated. A subcutaneous tunnel is made between the 2 incisions that must be wide enough, approximately 2 cm, to accommodate the ADQ muscle. The muscle is rotated 180° on its longitudinal axis, akin to turning a page in a book, with

addition to restoring opposition, it adds bulk to the thenar eminence and thereby improves the aesthetic appearance of the thumb. The ADQ transfer is also suitable for cases in which there is

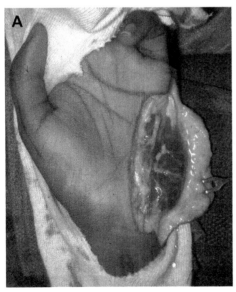
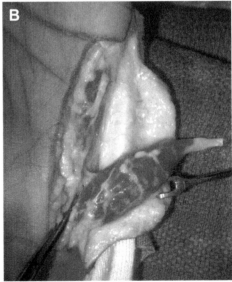

Fig. 10. (*A*) The entire length of the ADQ is exposed. (*B*) The muscle is detached distally, and care is taken to protect the neurovascular bundle (end of clamp). (*C*) The ADQ is passed through a wide subcutaneous tunnel. (*D*) The ADQ was attached to the insertion site of the APB; the muscle was pale as a result of being denervated.

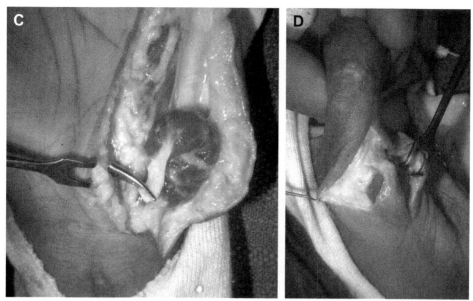

Fig. 10. (*Continued*)

the result that the original ulnar portion of the muscle is proximal and the original deep portion is superficial (**Figs. 10** and **11**). If necessary, the origin of the ADQ from the pisiform can be partially released to mobilize the muscle sufficiently to reach the thumb. The muscle origin can be completely released, but then its attachment to the FCU must be preserved to protect the neurovascular bundle

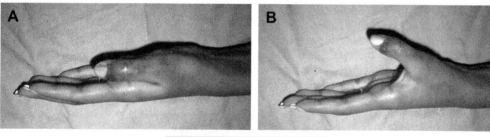

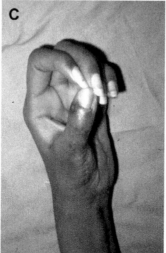

Fig. 11. Postoperative results. (*A*) No loss of adduction. (*B*) Full abduction restored. (*C*) Complete opposition.

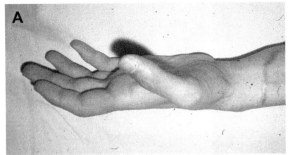

Fig. 12. A 35-year-old patient sustained lacerations of all flexor tendons and both median and ulnar nerves. (*A*) After tendon and nerve repairs, the patient regained satisfactory digital flexion and protective sensibility, but all intrinsic muscles remained paralyzed, an intrinsic minus hand. The ECRL was used as the motor for intrinsic transfers to the fingers, and clawing was eliminated. (*B*) Paralysis of the thenar muscles with no thumb abduction.

from any undue tension being placed on it.[33] Before suturing the tendon to the tendon of the APB, the tourniquet is released to evaluate the vascularity of the muscle. If it is pale in color, there is compression somewhere along its course through the subcutaneous tunnel or its neurovascular pedicle is twisted. Only after determining that muscle vascularity is not compromised is the tendon of the ADQ sutured to the tendon of the APB with the thumb flexed and pronated.

Extensor Carpi Ulnaris

In 1947, Phalen and Miller[16] described a procedure using the ECU for thumb opposition. For the tendon to reach the thumb, the investigators resorted to the method that Ney[11] proposed in 1921 of prolonging it with the tendon of an EPB that is transected at its musculotendinous junction and rerouted volarly. The insertion of the EPB into the dorsal base of the proximal phalanx of the thumb is left intact. Instead of rerouting the EPB through the carpal tunnel and attaching it to either the PL or FCR, which Ney recommended, Phalen and Miller rerouted the EPB tendon subcutaneously across the palm and attached it to the ECU that is transected at its insertion into the base of the fifth metacarpal.

An ECU opposition transfer requires 3 incisions (**Fig. 12**). The first is a longitudinal incision over the dorsoradial aspect of the forearm at the site where the APL and EPB cross the radial wrist extensors. The musculotendinous junction of the EIP is identified and transected proximal to the extensor retinaculum. A second incision is made over the dorsum of the thumb MP joint where the cut end of the EPB tendon is withdrawn. It is important to mobilize the intact portion of the EPB tendon up to the MP joint but not distal to it. If the portion is mobilized distal to the joint, it can shift volarly and become an MP flexor, and, if the portion is not dissected up to the joint, a reverse

deformity of MP hyperextension is likely to occur.[33] It is also important that the fascial connections between the EPB and EPL tendons are cut to avoid the transfer from hyperextending the IP joint. A third incision is made in a longitudinal manner on the ulnar side of the wrist and distal forearm where the ECU tendon, after it is transected at its insertion, is withdrawn proximal to the extensor retinaculum. A subcutaneous tunnel is made just proximal to the pisiform across the palm to the incision over the thumb MP joint. The EPB tendon is passed distally to proximally though the tunnel and sutured to the ECU tendon with the thumb in full opposition (**Figs. 13** and **14**). Occasionally, the EPB may be absent or hypoplastic, and, in such situations, a free tendon graft is necessary to prolong the ECU.

A prerequisite for a Phalen-Miller transfer is normal strength of the FCU muscle to preserve

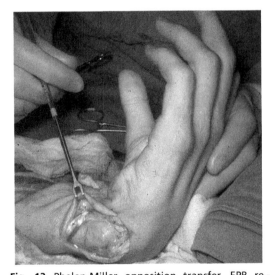

Fig. 13. Phalen-Miller opposition transfer. EPB rerouted across the palm of the hand and attached to the ECU that had been transected at its insertion.

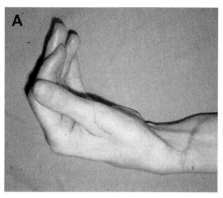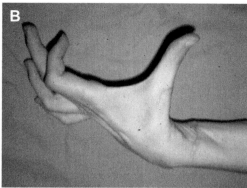

Fig. 14. (*A*) No loss of thumb adduction. (*B*) Excellent thumb abduction.

postoperative wrist balance.[16] When the transfer is performed in a patient with severe weakness or paralysis of the FCU, the postoperative result is a wrist that is radially deviated. Therefore, the procedure should not be performed in the patient with a high ulnar nerve injury that results in denervation of the FCU. However, it can be used for combined median and low ulnar nerve injuries as well as brachial plexus injuries when other potential donor tendons are either unavailable or are required for other transfers.

Palmaris Longus Transfer

A PL transfer for thumb opposition is commonly referred to as the Camitz procedure, named after the surgeon who described it in 1929.[15] The procedure is almost always performed in conjunction with decompression of the median nerve and usually when the nerve decompression is too late to restore intrinsic muscle function but not too late to relieve the patient's subjective sensory complaints.[37] However, some recommend the transfer in conjunction with a median decompression even when they expect that the thenar muscles will regain their strength. Their reasoning is that the operation is uncomplicated and adds

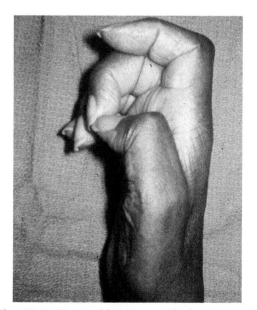

Fig. 15. A 60-year-old woman with chronic carpal tunnel of more than 5 years' duration. In addition to severe sensory complaints of nighttime paresthesias, there was complete thenar paralysis and atrophy.

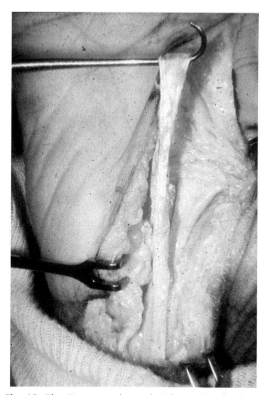

Fig. 16. The PL was prolonged with a strip of palmar fascia (pretendinous band).

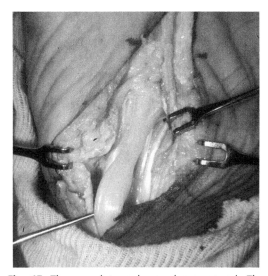

Fig. 17. The carpal tunnel was decompressed. The hour glass appearance of the median nerve reflected the chronicity of the compression.

little to the operative time.[26] A Camitz transfer restores thumb abduction but not pronation, and Smith referred to it as an "abductorplasty" rather than an opposition tendon transfer.[3] The procedure is not recommended for a traumatic median nerve laceration at the wrist level because the PL is likely to be damaged and scarred by the injury.

The PL is absent in approximately 20% of extremities and obviously it is important to determine that the muscle is present before proceeding with surgery.[3] This is determined by palpating for the tendon with the patient actively flexing the wrist against resistance and simultaneously opposing the tip of the thumb to the tip of the little finger. If the PL is present, a longitudinal incision is made in the palm beginning in the distal palmar

crease in line with the web space between the middle and ring fingers and continuing the incision proximally into the wrist flexion crease (**Fig. 15**). The incision is continued in the crease in an ulnar direction for a short distance and is then carried proximally in a longitudinal manner on the distal forearm for 2 to 3 cm. By curving the incision ulnarly in the wrist crease, injury to the palmar cutaneous branch of the median nerve is avoided and the risk of a postoperative scar contracture is reduced. The PL is identified in the distal forearm and is prolonged into the distal palm by preserving its continuity with a 1.5-cm-wide strip of palmar fascia, namely, the pretendinous band to either the middle or ring finger (**Fig. 16**). The transverse carpal ligament is divided and carpal tunnel decompressed (**Fig. 17**). A second incision is made over the dorsoradial side of the thumb MP joint, and a subcutaneous tunnel is made between this site and the PL tendon in the distal forearm. The tunnel must be sufficiently wide to permit easy passage of the PL tendon with its attached strip of palmar fascia. The end of that fascia strip is then sutured to the APB tendon with the wrist in neutral position and the thumb in full abduction (**Fig. 18**).

The advantages of the procedure are that there is no functional loss from using a PL tendon, and the operation is uncomplicated and requires only 2 incisions. It is an excellent procedure for the elderly patient with chronic carpal tunnel syndrome who has disabling thenar paralysis. Its main disadvantage is that the transfer essentially only abducts the thumb and does not restore either pronation or MP flexion (**Fig. 19**). An alternative method is to route the PL around the FCU and suture it to the proximal end of the EPB tendon that has been rerouted, similar to the technique used in the Phalen-Miller opposition transfer.[33]

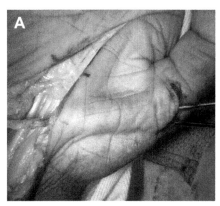
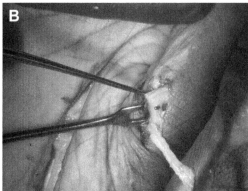

Fig. 18. (A) The PL and the attached fascia were passed subcutaneously to the radial side of the MP joint. (B) The end of the palmar fascia was sutured to the tendon of the APB.

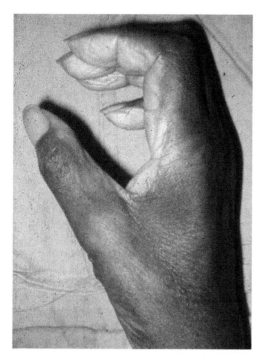

Fig. 19. Postoperative thumb abduction was restored; even some pronation was restored.

When any of these 5 procedures cannot be performed because of trauma resulting in a serious neurologic deficit with severe scarring or a progressive neurologic disorder, less commonly used transfers may be effective.

Extensor Digiti Quinti Proprius Transfer

An EDQP transfer is similar to an EIP transfer, but there is a significant difference in the anatomy of the extensor tendons to the index and little fingers. Both fingers have 2 extensor tendons, an EDC and a proprius that for the index is the EIP and for the little finger is the EDQP. This is where the similarity ends. Although both extensors are almost always present in the index finger and each can completely extend the finger, the same is not as true in the little finger. The EDQP is the far more constant tendon; the EDC is often poorly developed, and its ability to extend the MP joint depends on its junctura tendinum connection to the ring finger, which is often poorly developed. If the EDQP was used as a transfer in such situations, the result would be a loss of extension of the little finger. Therefore, the important prerequisite for an EDQP opposition transfer is to first determine that the EDC tendon to the finger is present and that it can completely extend the MP joint. This is determined at surgery by placing traction on the tendon. Another potential problem

is that the EDQP tendon is not of sufficient length to reach the insertion site on the thumb unless it is prolonged with a strip of the extensor hood. However, even with a careful repair of the hood, an extension lag at the MP joint is a common occurrence.[22]

Extensor Carpi Radialis Longus, Extensor Carpi Radialis Brevis, Extensor Carpi Ulnaris, and Brachioradialis Transfers

In 1962, Henderson[19] published an article on the use of the 3 wrist extensors (ECRL, ECRB, and ECU) and the BR as transfers for restoring thumb opposition. The ECU transfer was essentially identical to that reported by Phalen and Miller[16] 15 years earlier in 1947. Henderson recommended use of an ECRL, an ECRB, or a BR when wrist and finger flexors were required for other transfers or were unsuitable to transfer because of marked weakness and/or scarring. Of these 3 muscles, either of the radial wrist extensors, the ECRL or ECRB, gave the best results. The selected tendon is routed around the ulnar border of the wrist and prolonged with a free tendon graft that is passed subcutaneously across the palm and inserted into the tendon of the APB. Instead of prolonging the wrist extensor with a free tendon graft, it can be attached to the EPB tendon, which is cut at its musculotendinous junction and routed across the palm, similar to the Phalen-Miller transfer. Attaching the wrist extensor to the EPL that is rerouted across the palm has also been recommended.[38] The BR was the least effective motor in Henderson's series. However, it should be considered when other motors are unavailable.

Flexor Pollicis Longus and Extensor Pollicis Longus Transfers

When there is total or near-total paralysis of all the intrinsic muscles in the thumb (intrinsic minus thumb), which occurs in combined low median and ulnar nerve palsies, the intact extrinsic FPL and EPL muscles produce a thumb deformity characterized by adduction, supination, MP hyperextension, and IP flexion. The FPL and EPL are attempting to substitute for the absent intrinsics. The adduction component of the thumb deformity is caused by the EPL, which by virtue of its path around the Lister tubercle courses dorsal to the TM joint in the coronal plane and is therefore an adductor of the thumb as well as an extensor. It is for that reason that thumb adduction is still possible, although not with great force, when the main adductor of the digit, the intrinsic adductor pollicis, is paralyzed. The FPL in its course through the carpal canal and then through the flexor sheath in the digit passes over the middle of the TM joint and is neither an abductor nor an adductor of the joint. Its function is essentially thumb flexion. Because all the intrinsic thumb muscles (with the exception of the opponens pollicis) insert on the base of the proximal phalanx and into the dorsal extensor hood (intrinsics innervated by the median nerve on the radial side and intrinsics innervated by the ulnar nerve on the ulnar side), they are flexors of the MP joint and extensors of the IP joint. The intrinsic and extrinsic thumb muscles balance each other, and, when intrinsic muscle function is lost, the MP joint hyperextends (provided it can passively do so) and the IP joint flexes. The IP flexion is usually severe and is commonly referred to as hyperflexion.[26,33] The hyperflexion is the attempt by the FPL and EPL to provide for effective grasp in the absence of intrinsic muscle function. However, the grasp is ineffective because the IP hyperflexion prevents the thumb pulp from contacting the index finger for either tip-to-tip pulp pinch or for side key pinch. Instead, the thumbnail or, even worse, the dorsum of the distal segment of the thumb comes in contact with the fingers. Usually, the patient is still capable of grasping objects between the side of the thumb and the radial side of the palm. That grasp may be sufficient for most activities, and a tendon transfer is unnecessary. However, when the patient has a significant disability, grasp can usually be improved using either the FPL or the EPL as a tendon transfer or, in some cases, both tendons. For this reason, FPL and EPL transfers are discussed together.

An FPL transfer is generally used for the patient with an intrinsic minus thumb and a severe and fixed flexion deformity of the IP joint. The objectives of the operation are to relieve the deforming force of the FPL on the IP joint and to enhance the force of thumb pinch to the fingers. The objective is not to restore thumb pronation. At surgery, the insertion of the FPL tendon is released from its insertion into the base of the distal phalanx. It is then retrieved through an incision on the volar aspect of the wrist and rerouted using any of the variety of techniques previously described. The IP joint is commonly arthrodesed in extension to permit good contact of the thumb pulp with the fingers. Patients who have had the transfer together with an IP fusion seem to sense that they now have a functioning short flexor muscle and they are no longer dependent on the EPL to adduct their thumbs. Instead, the EPL reverts to its more normal function of moving the thumb away from the fingers. The FPL that Burkhalter[29] referred to as "the new FPB" now provides effective grasp.

Mangus[23] modified the procedure by routing the FPL around the FCU and then subcutaneously across the palm. Instead of arthrodesing the IP joint, Mangus tenodesed the joint with the distal remnant of the FPL that he preserved when the tendon was transected. His modification resembles the Bunnell technique for an FDS opposition transfer in that the FPL changes direction near the pisiform and follows the course of the APB rather than the Royle-Thompson technique in which the tendon curves more distally in the palm around the ulna border of the palmar fascia and then takes a transverse course across the palm in line with the radial head of the FPB. The Royle-Thompson procedure is generally preferred for the total intrinsic minus thumb. Although restoring some pronation to the thumb is beneficial, it is more important to restore the force of flexion.

The FPL has also been used in a manner that leaves it intact throughout its length, including its insertion. Makin transferred the FPL in continuity through an oblique osteotomy in the proximal phalanx.[20] The FPL tendon spirals around the phalanx and MP joint. The osteotomy is then fixed with a longitudinal Kirschner wire, which also stabilizes the IP joint in extension. Oberlin and Alnot[39] used a similar technique, but, rather than transferring the FPL through an osteotomy, they transferred it through either the IP or the MP joint, which was then arthrodesed. Oberlin and Alnot emphasized the importance of the FPL passing over the dorsal surface of the MP joint and not over the dorsal surface of the proximal phalanx.

In some cases, the FPL is too weak to be used as a transfer, yet the flexion contracture of the IP joint can be as severe. The contracture is secondary to the tenodesis of the joint by the FPL, which develops from an overactive EPL that extends and supinates the TM and MP joints.[33] An EPL opposition transfer can sometimes correct the deformity, provided the EPL is under voluntary control. If the muscle is spastic, the transfer would result in the thumb positioned in front of the fingers, which would interfere with their function. In such situations, the patient is usually unable to actively extend and abduct the thumb because the APL is not strong enough to overcome the spastic EPL. When there is voluntary control of the EPL, the technique for transfer first involves releasing the tendon from its insertion into the distal phalanx and then from the radial and ulnar portions of the extensor hood over the proximal phalanx and MP joint. Through a second incision over the middorsum of the wrist and forearm, the EPL tendon is retrieved proximal to the extensor retinaculum and its muscle belly is freed more proximally. A third incision is made on the ulnar side of the wrist near the pisiform. The EPL is routed to this site and then subcutaneously across the palm to the initial incision on the dorsum of the thumb. The MP joint is arthrodesed, the EPL tendon is looped around the radial and ulnar portions of the extensor hood, and the tendon is sutured to itself with the thumb in full opposition and the wrist in approximately 30° flexion, similar to the positions in previously described opposition transfers. The radial and ulnar portions of the extensor mechanism are then sutured together, thereby preserving extension of the IP joint. At surgery, after the transfer with the wrist in neutral position, the fingers should clear the thumb. This is important because the only remaining muscles that can extend the thumb are the APL and EPB, and there is no assurance that they are strong enough to do so.

A modification of the procedure has been recommended in which the EPL passes through a window in the interosseous membrane rather than around the ulnar side of the wrist and an MP arthrodesis is not included.[40,41] Although good results were reported, the line of pull of the EPL does not achieve as much thumb abduction as when the tendon is routed around the ulnar side of the wrist, and routing the tendon through the interosseous membrane adds the risk of adhesions at that site, which can restrict postoperative tendon gliding.[33]

EPL opposition transfers are usually reserved for patients with significant and progressive neurologic problems such as syringomyelia and Charcot-Marie-Tooth disease.

SUMMARY

Opposition is not grasp but a preposition for grasp that involves 3 components of thumb movements: abduction, flexion, and pronation. The muscles that provide these movements are the intrinsic muscles in the thenar eminence: the APB, FPB (particularly the radial head), and opponens pollicis. The most important muscle is the APB for which the direction of pull is toward the pisiform. The other intrinsic thumb muscle that is not in the thenar eminence is the adductor pollicis, which, as its name indicates, is a thumb adductor and provides forceful pinch, either tip-to-tip pinch to a finger or key pinch to the side of the index finger. The extrinsic EPL also adducts the thumb but not with the same force as the adductor pollicis. Thumb opposition is usually lost with paralysis of the thenar muscles innervated by the median nerve. However, in many patients, thumb abduction remains because the radial head of the FPB has a dual innervation through the ulnar nerve.

Many opposition transfers have been described that differ in the donor tendon (or muscle when the ADQ is used), route of transfer, and method of attachment to the thumb. No one transfer is applicable for every clinical condition, and each transfer has its advantages and disadvantages. Many factors must be evaluated to decide if surgery is likely to be beneficial and then to decide the optimum treatment.

REFERENCES

1. Jacob B, Thompson TC. Opposition of the thumb and its restoration. J Bone Joint Surg Am 1960;42: 1015–26.
2. Bunnell S. Opposition of the thumb. J Bone Joint Surg 1938;20:269–84.
3. Smith RJ. Tendon transfers of the hand and forearm. Boston: Little Brown; 1987. p. 57–83.
4. Rowntree T. Anomalous innervation of the hand muscles. J Bone Joint Surg Br 1949;31:505–10.
5. Steindler A. Orthopaedic operations on the hand. JAMA 1918;71:1288.
6. Krukenberg H. Uber ersatz des M. opponens pollicis. Z Orthop Clin 1922;42:178 [in German].
7. Royle ND. An operation for paralysis of the intrinsic muscles of the thumb. JAMA 1938;111:612–3.
8. Thompson TC. A modified operation for opponens paralysis. J Bone Joint Surg 1942;24:632–40.
9. Huber E. Hilfsoperation bet median uhlahmung. Dtsch Arch Klin Med 1921;136:271 [in German].
10. Nicolaysen J. Transplantation des m. abductor dig V. die fenlander oppositions fehigkeit des daumens. Dtsch Z Chir 1922;168:133 [in German].
11. Ney KW. A tendon transplant for intrinsic hand muscle paralysis. Surg Gynecol Obstet 1921;33:342–8.
12. Taylor RT. Reconstruction of the hand. Surg Gynecol Obstet 1921;32:237–48.
13. Lyle HH. Results of an operation for thenar paralysis of the thumb (extensor-flexor-flexorplasty). Ann Surg 1924;79:933.
14. Howell BW. A new operation for opponens paralysis of the thumb. Lancet 1926;16:131.
15. Camitz H. Surgical treatment of paralysis of opponens muscle of thumbs. Acta Chir Scand 1929;65:77–81.
16. Phalen GS, Miller RC. The transfer of wrist extensor muscles to restore or reinforce flexion of power of the fingers and opposition the thumb. J Bone Joint Surg 1947;29:993–7.
17. Zancolli E. Cirugia de la mano. Musculos intrinsecos. Prensa Med Argent 1956;43:1299 [in German].
18. Riordan DC. Surgery of the paralytic hand. In: Reynolds FC, editor, American Academy of Orthopaedic Surgeons instructional course lectures, vol. 16. St Louis (MO): Mosby; 1959. p. 79–90.
19. Henderson ED. Transfer of wrist extensors and brachioradialis to restore opposition of the thumb. J Bone Joint Surg 1962;44:513–22.
20. Makin M. Translocation of the flexor pollicis longus tendon to restore opposition. J Bone Joint Surg Br 1967;49:458–61.

21. Tubiana R, Valentin P. Opposition of the thumb. Surg Clin North Am 1968;48:967.
22. Schneider LH. Opponensplasty using the extensor digiti minimi. J Bone Joint Surg 1969;51:1297–302.
23. Mangus DJ. Flexor pollicis longus tendon transfer for restoration of thumb opposition. Plast Reconstr Surg 1973;52:155–9.
24. Burkhalter W, Christensen RC, Brown P. Extensor indicis proprius opponensplasty. J Bone Joint Surg Am 1973;55:725–32.
25. North ER, Littler JW. Transferring the flexor superficialis tendon. Technical considerations in the prevention of proximal interphalangeal joint disability. J Hand Surg 1980;5:498–501.
26. Davis TR, Barton NJ. Median nerve palsy. In: Green DP, Hotchkiss RN, Pederson WC, editors. Green's operative hand surgery. 4th edition. New York: Churchill Livingstone; 1999. p. 1497–525.
27. Cooney WP, Linscheid RL, An KN. Opposition of the thumb: an anatomic and biomechanical study of tendon transfers. J Hand Surg Am 1984;9:777–86.
28. Braun RM. Palmaris longus tendon transfer for augmentation of the thenar musculature in low median palsy. J Hand Surg 1978;3:488–91.
29. Burkhalter WE. In: Green DP, editor. Operative hand surgery. 2nd edition. New York: Churchill Livingstone; 1988. p. 1515–25.
30. Littler JW, Cooley SG. Opposition of the thumb and its restoration by abductor digiti quinti transfer. J Bone Joint Surg 1963;45:1389–96.
31. Imbriglia JE, Hadberg WC, Baratz ME. Median nerve reconstruction. In: Peimer CA, editor. Surgery of the hand and upper extremity. New York: McGraw-Hill; 1996. p. 1381–97.
32. Burkhalter W. Early tendon transfer in upper extremity peripheral nerve injury. Clin Orthop 1974; 104:68–9.
33. Berger RA, Weiss AP. Hand surgery, vol I. New York: Lippincott Williams & Wilkins; 2004. p. 959–78.
34. Anderson GA, Lee V, Sundararaj GD. Opponensplasty by extensor indicis and flexor digitorum superficialis tendon transfer. J Hand Surg Br 1992;17: 611–4.
35. Brown EZ, Teague MA, Snyder CC. Prevention of extensor lag after extensor indicis proprius tendon transfer. J Hand Surg 1979;4:168–72.
36. Calandruccio JH, Jobe MT. Paralytic hand. In: Canale ST, editor. Campbell's operative orthopaedics, Chapter 68, 10th edition. St Louis (MO): Mosby; 2003. p. 3628–33.
37. Littler JW, Li CS. Primary restoration of thumb opposition with median nerve compression. Plast Reconstr Surg 1967;39:74–5.
38. Kaplan I, Dinner M, Chait L. Use of extensor pollicis longus tendon as a distal extension for an opposition transfer. Plast Reconstr Surg 1976;57:186–90.
39. Oberlin C, Alnot JY. Opponensplasty through translocation of the flexor pollicis longus. Techniques and indications. Ann Chir Main 1988;7:25–31.
40. Mennen U. Extensor pollicis longus opposition transfer. J Hand Surg Am 1922;17:809–11.
41. Moutet F, Frere G, Massart P. Reanimation of thumb opposition by the extensor pollicis longus. Report of sixteen cases. Ann Chir Main 1986;5:36–41.

Restoration of Pinch in Intrinsic Muscles of the Hand

Steve K. Lee, MD[a], Jamie R. Wisser, MD[b,c],*

KEYWORDS

• Restoration • Pinch • Intrinsic muscles • Hand

One of the integral functions of the intrinsic muscles is thumb to index finger key and tip pinch. This function is important for many activities of daily living such as using keys, holding eating utensils, getting dressed (buttons and zippers), holding a toothbrush, opening small caps, and tearing open packages. The intrinsic muscles primarily involved in this action are the adductor pollicis (AP) muscle, the first dorsal interosseous (DI) muscle, and the flexor pollicis brevis (FPB) muscle.

ANATOMY
AP Muscle

The AP muscle is composed of 2 heads: transverse and oblique. Both heads are innervated by the motor branch of the ulnar nerve as the nerve passes between the 2 heads. The radial artery also passes between the 2 heads of the AP, from dorsal to palmar, to become the deep arch. The transverse head of the AP is broad and originates from the palmar aspect of the third metacarpal bone and inserts on the ulnar aspect of the thumb proximal phalanx base along with the oblique AP head and the deep head of the FPB. The oblique head originates from the palmar aspects of the second and third metacarpal bones, the capitate bone, the intercarpal ligaments, and the flexor carpi radialis (FCR) sheath. It inserts on the ulnar aspect of the thumb proximal phalanx base via a conjoint tendon that passes through the ulnar

sesamoid bone of the thumb metacarpophalangeal (MP) joint. The action of the muscle is to bring the thumb back to the plane of the palm and it is assisted by the FPB and the opponens pollicis.[1]

First DI Muscle

The first DI muscle is bipennate and originates on both the radial side of the second metacarpal bone and the proximal ulnar portion of the first metacarpal bone. It inserts on the radial aspect of the index finger proximal phalanx base and the index finger dorsal tendinous hood. The radial artery passes between the 2 heads as it courses from dorsal to palmar. Innervation of the first DI is the ulnar nerve. Its action is to abduct the index finger from the middle finger and assist the lumbricals in MP joint flexion and interphalangeal (IP) joint extension.[1]

FPB Muscle

The FPB has 2 heads: superficial and deep. The superficial head originates from the trapezium bone and the distal edge of the transverse carpal ligament. It inserts on the radial aspect of the thumb proximal phalanx base through the radial sesamoid bone of the thumb MP joint. The deep head is smaller and originates from the ulnar palmar portion of the first metacarpal bone and inserts on the ulnar aspect of the thumb proximal phalanx base along with the conjoint tendon of the transverse and oblique heads of the AP

[a] Hand and Upper Extremity Surgery Service, Hospital for Special Surgery, Weill Cornell Medical College, 535 East 70th Street, New York, NY 10021, USA
[b] Department of Orthopaedic Surgery, Division of Hand Surgery, NYU/Langone Medical Center, 550 1st Avenue, New York, NY 10016, USA
[c] Princeton Surgical Specialties, PA, 300B Princeton Hightstown Road, Suite 101, East Windsor, NJ 08520, USA
* Corresponding author. Princeton Surgical Specialties, PA, 300B Princeton Hightstown Road, Suite 101, East Windsor, NJ 08520, USA.
E-mail address: wisser4@comcast.net

Hand Clin 28 (2012) 45–51
doi:10.1016/j.hcl.2011.10.002
0749-0712/12/$ – see front matter © 2012 Elsevier Inc. All rights reserved.

muscle. The superficial head is innervated by the motor branch of the median nerve, and the deep head is innervated by the deep motor branch of the ulnar nerve. The action of the FPB is to flex the thumb MP joint.[1]

PATHOANATOMY

Loss of AP, FPB, and first DI muscle function results in weakness of thumb adduction, thumb MP flexion, and index finger MP stabilization. The patient feels that there is weakness of thumb key and tip pinch, among other activities of daily living stated earlier. Biomechanical studies suggest that up to 80% loss of power pinch occurs in patients with ulnar nerve palsy.[2] In cases of complete ulnar nerve palsy, the only adductor of the thumb remaining is the extensor pollicis longus (EPL)[3]; however, the remaining adduction is weak. If the joints are lax, contraction of the EPL, extensor pollicis brevis (EPB), and flexor pollicis longus (FPL) without the balancing action of the intrinsic muscles results in a concertina Z deformity of the thumb with MP hyperextension and IP joint flexion. Physical examination displays the telltale Froment sign: when the patient attempts to perform key pinch, the IP joint actively flexes as the patient uses the anterior interosseous nerve–innervated FPL to compensate for the lack of the AP, first DI, and portion of FPB function. The Jeanne sign is present if there is MP joint hyperextension.

ETIOLOGY

Several diseases or injuries can adversely affect a person's ability to initiate or generate pinch with adequate strength. Altered anatomy of the thumb or index finger due to trauma, congenital anomalies, degenerative and inflammatory joint disease, or extrinsic muscle/tendon abnormalities can adversely affect pinching mechanics.

Intrinsic muscle weakness affecting pinch primarily occurs as a result of disease involving the ulnar nerve. Most common neural causes include high or low crush injuries, partial or complete nerve laceration, brachial plexus injuries affecting ulnar nerve function, advanced ulnar nerve compression syndromes, cerebral vascular disease, or brain injury. Atypical causes of intrinsic muscle weakness include ulnar artery aneurysms and neuromuscular diseases, such as spastic cerebral palsy creating a thumb in palm deformity.

TREATMENT

When weakness is debilitating, then surgical management may be considered after the patient has completed a course of hand therapy and exercises to optimize compensating muscles. Hand therapy may consist of use of the EPL for adduction and FPL thumb flexion toward the index finger for pinch. Splints to stabilize the thumb MP joint and adaptive devices such as thicker handles for grasp during activities of daily living may be helpful. The goals of reconstructive surgery are to restore thumb adduction, stabilize the index finger MP joint so that the index finger is not pushed ulnarward by the thumb when pinching, and to stabilize the thumb MP and IP joints. Surgical management falls in 3 distinct categories: (1) augmentation of the AP muscle, (2) augmentation of the first DI muscle, and (3) stabilization of the thumb and index finger.

Augmentation of the AP Muscle

The need to restore the AP muscle during key or tip pinch requires use of a strong motor, such as the extensor carpi radialis brevis (ECRB), brachioradialis, flexor digitorum superficialis (FDS) III or IV, extensor indicis proprius (EIP), or extensor digiti quinti. Critical to any muscle tendon transfer to restore adductor function is the ability to maximize excursion, properly set tension, and use a functional pulley with as simple a direction of pull as possible.

Transfer techniques using wrist extensor motors require tendon lengthening with a tendon autograft, such as palmaris longus (PL), half of FCR, EIP, plantaris, or extensor digitorum longus donors. There is a trade-off between taking advantage of wrist extensor motor power and needing to use a tendon graft.

The choice between techniques should be based on several clinical factors. Patient demand, age, intact donor motor innervation, and the presence or absence of any associated functional deficits are critical in selecting a donor motor tendon unit. The main advantage of selecting a wrist extensor as a donor motor is that wrist extension and pinch are synergistic actions. Extrinsic digital extensors are weaker than superficial extrinsic digital flexors, and neither is as strong as a wrist extensor donor. The benefit of using an extrinsic digital motor is the ability to perform direct transfer without tendon graft. The trade-off is related to the amount of pinch strength that can be restored.

ECRB to AP muscle tendon transfer (lengthened via tendon graft)
Whether using the ECRB, the extensor carpi radialis longus as described by Solonen and Bakalim,[4] the extensor carpi ulnaris using the distal ulna as a pulley or brachioradialis as described by Boyes,[5] all thumb adductor tendon transfers using a wrist extensor donor requires a tendon graft extension.

Of the wrist extensor procedures, use of the ECRB as the donor motor source is effective in maximizing pinch strength with minimal donor site morbidity.

Surgical technique

An S-shaped incision is made between the second and third metacarpal bases. The ECRB insertion is released off the third metacarpal bone. A second incision is made proximal to dorsal wrist extensor retinaculum, and the ECRB tendon is pulled out of this wound. A third incision is made at the ulnar base of the thumb MP joint. Free tendon autograft (ie, PL if present, half of FCR if not) is passed from the thumb wound between the AP and interossei volar to the second metacarpal bone and dorsally out between the second and third metacarpal bones. The free graft is sutured to the AP tendon at its insertion. The wrist is held in neutral with the thumb placed adducted to the index finger. The proximal end of the tendon graft is passed through the ECRB tendon in the Pulvertaft method and tension set with the ECRB distracted to mid-excursion length. The mid-excursion length is determined by marking the ECRB at its resting position, then pulling the tendon distally to its maximum excursion and marking this point. The mid-excursion length is halfway between these 2 marks. The tendon graft is passed through the ECRB at this mid-excursion point and held with a single suture. Passively flexing and extending the wrist enables thumb abduction/adduction

tension to be assessed. Once proper tension has been achieved, the tendon graft is Pulvertaft woven 3 times through the ECRB tendon (**Figs. 1** and **2**).

The thumb is immobilized in a static thumb spica splint or cast for 4 weeks postoperatively. A custom forearm-based thumb spica thermoplastic splint in a functional position is then made by a hand therapist and gentle active and active assist range of motion exercises are initiated. Resistive pinch and grip strengthening is begun at the eighth postoperative week. All but the most high-demand activities can be resumed 3 months postoperatively, with return to all levels of unrestricted activity at 6 months postoperatively. The patient is instructed to wear a protective thumb spica splint until 1 year postoperatively when engaging in high-risk activities, such as snow skiing.

FDS III or IV to AP muscle tendon transfer

Using extrinsic digital flexors to recreate thumb adduction is an equally popular transfer procedure. One major advantage of the FDS transfer is that the operation is limited to the palmar structures within the hand; another advantage is that direct tendon transfer may be performed without a tendon graft.

Either the middle finger or ring finger FDS may be used in low ulnar nerve palsy[6]; only the middle finger FDS should be used in cases of upper ulnar nerve palsy because the ring finger flexor

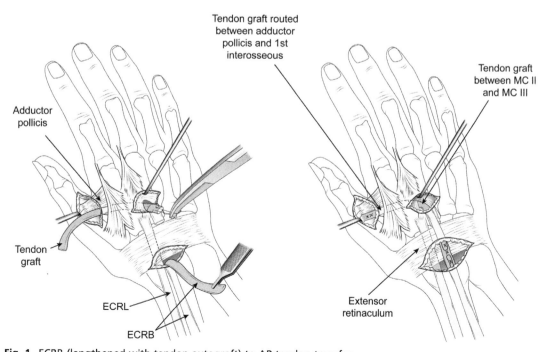

Tendon graft routed between adductor pollicis and 1st interosseous

Tendon graft between MC II and MC III

Adductor pollicis

Tendon graft

ECRL

ECRB

Extensor retinaculum

Fig. 1. ECRB (lengthened with tendon autograft) to AP tendon transfer.

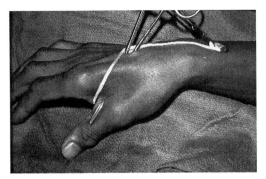

Fig. 2. ECRB (lengthened with tendon autograft) to AP tendon transfer.

digitorum profundus (FDP) function is weak or absent in upper ulnar nerve palsy. Despite the theoretical advantage of increased excursion and pinch strength with the use of the ring finger FDS tendon as the donor, the middle finger FDS tendon has the advantages of (1) not presenting an issue with high ulnar nerve lesions with a weak or absent FDP to the ring finger and (2) greater tendon length allowing the harvest to be proximal to the decussation. This situation minimizes the chance of developing a secondary swan-neck deformity, particularly in the patient with ligamentous laxity. Preserving the decussation reduces the chance of hindering FDP motion by loose FDS tails in the sheath. The FDS is harvested through an oblique skin incision just palmar to the MP joint. The A1 pulley is released and the FDS tendon is pulled

out of the wound, visualizing the decussation. The tendon is transected just proximal to the decussation.[7] The pulley for the tendon transfer is the vertical septum of the superficial palmar fascia attached to the second metacarpal when the middle finger FDS is used as the donor.

An incision is made on the ulnar side of the thumb MP joint. The FDS tendon is then tunneled subcutaneously toward the AP tendon insertion. The tendon graft is then sutured to the AP tendon insertion, with the tension set with the wrist held in 30° of extension with the thumb adducted to the index finger (**Figs. 3** and **4**).

EIP to AP muscle tendon transfer
The EIP is lengthened with a free tendon graft. The graft is then passed from dorsal to palmar between the second and third metacarpal bones and routed toward the AP tendon as in the ECRB to AP technique.[7] The donor defect in the extensor hood is carefully repaired, with the distal remnant stump of the donor tendon being tenodesed to the remaining index extrinsic extensor to reduce the risk of a secondary extensor lag.

Authors' preferred method for adductor functional restoration
Our preference is the ECRB to AP transfer given the synergistic wrist tenodesis action. If there is radial nerve palsy and the FDP to the middle finger is intact, then the middle finger FDS to the AP is preferred.

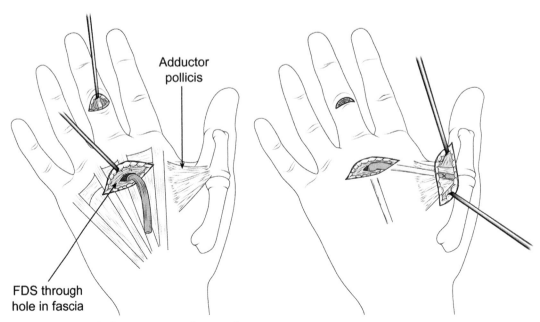

Adductor pollicis

FDS through hole in fascia

Fig. 3. FDS of middle finger to AP tendon transfer.

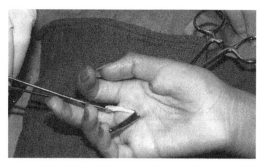

Fig. 4. FDS of middle finger to AP tendon transfer.

Augmentation of the First DI Muscle

To augment the first DI muscle, several tendon transfers have been described: (1) abductor pollicis longus (APL), (2) EIP, (3) PL, others (EPB, FDS).

APL to first DI muscle tendon transfer

One slip of the APL is detached from its insertion on the first metacarpal bone. The slip is transferred proximally out of the first compartment pulley and passed subcutaneously toward the first DI tendon. The APL slip must be lengthened with a free tendon graft, such as PL autograft. The tendon graft is sutured to the first DI tendon insertion site distally. It is important to suture the tendon autograft palmar to the axis of rotation of the MP joint. Proximally the tendon autograft is interwoven into the transferred APL slip via the Pulvertaft method (**Figs. 5** and **6**).[8] The graft is tensioned with the index finger abducted maximally and the APL at half maximal excursion as stated in the section on ECRB to AP transfer. Nemoto[9] reported satisfactory results with transfer in a 2-patient case report, but Fischer and colleagues[10] believed that the transfer gave limited results in a series of 9 patients. The mean force of index finger abduction was 58% of the unaffected side. Mean key pinch was 73% of the unaffected side.

EIP to first DI muscle tendon transfer

The EIP is approached distally. The tendon is extended, with a strip of the index finger extensor hood and divided. The extensor hood is repaired and the distal EIP stump is tenodesed to the extensor digitorum communis. The EIP is brought proximally to the wrist level through a small incision. The EIP is then passed subcutaneously to the first DI tendon and sutured to it palmar to the axis of rotation of the MP joint.[11] Originally described by Brand,[12] the usefulness of this technique has been disputed. Because the direction of pull is ulnar to the index finger MP joint and not radial, Neviaser and colleagues[8] consider this transfer inadequate and unsatisfactory.

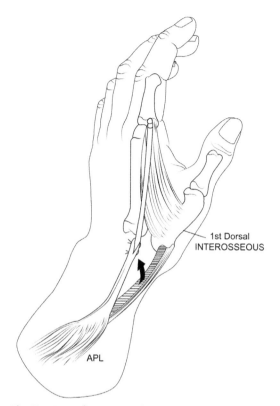

Fig. 5. APL to first DI muscle tendon transfer.

PL to first DI muscle tendon transfer

The PL tendon is lengthened through the palmar fascia as in the Camitz procedure. It is then transferred subcutaneously to the thumb and sutured to the first DI tendon palmar to the index finger MP joint axis of rotation.[13] As in the original Camitz procedure for abductor pollicis brevis augmentation, this transfer probably acts more as a tenodesis than active tendon transfer for index finger MP abduction.

Other transfers to augment the first DI muscle

Other donors that have been described are the EPB[14] (**Fig. 7**) and ring finger FDS.[15] Nobuta and colleagues[16] reported on 16 EPB to first DI

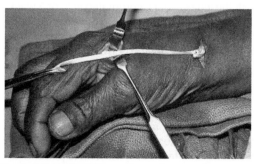

Fig. 6. APL to first DI muscle tendon transfer.

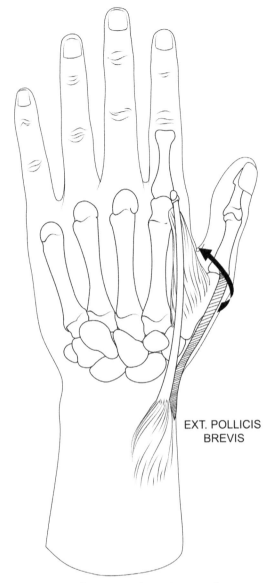

EXT. POLLICIS
BREVIS

Fig. 7. EPB to first DI muscle tendon transfer.

transfers with satisfactory results. Postoperatively, all of these transfers require immobilization in a forearm-based radial gutter thumb spica splint with the index finger incorporated in it for 3 weeks. The wrist is placed in 10° of extension. The index finger MP joint is placed in 30° of flexion and 20° of abduction. The thumb is in a functional position.

Authors' preferred method for augmentation of the first DI muscle

Transfer of an APL slip is our preferred method. There is usually a sufficient slip available as a donor, the vector of pull is appropriate, the transfer is surgically technically efficient to perform, and the results to stabilize the index MP joint are

generally satisfactory. The slip to harvest is generally the second widest; we leave the widest slip for its native function. We use the PL tendon to lengthen the tendon or half of the FCR tendon if the PL is absent.

Joint Stabilization

In clinical cases in which thumb or index joint instability limit motor tendon transfer effectiveness or in cases of joint arthrosis, joint arthrodesis may be indicated. Soft tissue joint stabilizing procedures remain an alternative, but are less predictable in restoring and preserving joint stability and may be contraindicated in patients with heavy-demand occupations.

Arthrodesis techniques for the MP or IP joints of the thumb and index finger are designed to maintain as much digital length as possible, preserve functional joint angles, use fixation techniques to create immediate stability and maximize bone contact between decorticated joint surfaces to promote union. There are a few described arthrodesis techniques, including cup and cone decortications and straight osteotomies. Fixation alternatives include Kirschner wire (K-wire) fixation, tension band fixation, plate and screws, and headless compression screws. K-wire fixation is performed with at least 2 crossing K-wires using 0.035 or 0.045 inch K-wires that are cut beneath the skin because they are to remain in place until radiographic signs of union occur. Tension band fixation is performed with 2 K-wires placed parallel followed by a 24-gauge or 26-gauge figure-of-8 tension band wire (**Figs. 8 and 9**). Rigid plate fixation provides immediate stability, allowing for early digital mobility and strengthening. A low-profile locking or nonlocking plate is positioned slightly radial to the dorsal central line to reduce the risk of secondary EPL tendonitis.

Arthrodesis of the MP joint

Arthrodesis of the MP joint of the thumb is performed with the MP joint placed at 20° of flexion and slight pronation. Arthrodesis of the index MP

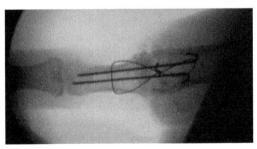

Fig. 8. Thumb MP arthrodesis with tension band technique (anterior posterior radiographic view).

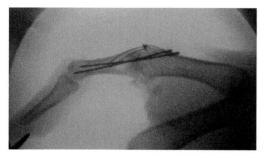

Fig. 9. Thumb MP arthrodesis with tension band technique (lateral radiographic view).

joint is performed with the MP joint positioned at 35° to 40° of flexion, 5° to 10° of radial inclination, and slight supination to enhance index to thumb tip contact. Arthrodeses of these joints is considered in cases of severe joint laxity or in cases of joint arthrosis.

Arthrodesis of the IP joint
When fusing the IP joint of the thumb, 15° of flexion and slight pronation is the fixation position of choice. Index finger proximal interphalangeal (PIP) joint arthrodesis is performed at 35° to 40° of flexion and 5° of supination. The position of distal interphalangeal (DIP) joint arthrodesis should be 10° to 15° of flexion and 5° of supination to enhance index fingertip contact with the thumb.

Authors' preferred arthrodesis method
Cup and cone decortication grants the largest degree of freedom to orient the joint before fixation. After fixation, if the joint position is incorrect, simple removal of the K-wire, reorientation of the join, and replacement of the K-wires is performed. K-wire/tension band fixation is preferred for MP joints and K-wire fixation is preferred for PIP and DIP joints. PIP joint fixation is achieved by first placing 1 K-wire from proximal to distal in the middle phalanx obliquely, reducing the joint, then driving it back retrograde into the proximal phalanx. A second K-wire is driven from proximal to distal longitudinally down the center of the joint. For DIP joint fixation, 2 K-wires are placed from proximal to distal in the distal phalanx and out the fingertip. The joint is reduced and the K-wires are driven back retrograde into the middle phalanx.

SUMMARY

The primary muscles responsible for key and tip pinch are the AP and first DI muscles. Numerous conditions can lead to their dysfunction, the most common being ulnar neuropathy. Nonoperative treatment consists of exercises of the compensating EPL and FPL muscles and adaptive devices with larger grips. If these measures fail, tendon transfers may be used. The most common tendon transfer sets are the ECRB to AP tendon transfer and the APL to first DI tendon transfer, both requiring free tendon grafts to lengthen the donor muscle/tendon unit. In cases of joint instability or arthrosis, arthrodesis of thumb and index finger joints may be indicated.

REFERENCES

1. Platzer W. 5th edition. Color atlas of human anatomy, vol 1. Stuttgart (Germany): Thieme; 2004.
2. Goldner JL. Tendon transfers for irreparable peripheral nerve injuries of the upper extremity. Orthop Clin N Am 1974;5(2):343–75.
3. Smith RJ. Extensor carpi radialis brevis tendon transfer for thumb adduction–a study of power pinch. J Hand Surg Am 1983;8(1):4–15.
4. Solonen KA, Bakalim GE. Restoration of pinch grip in traumatic ulnar palsy. Hand 1976;8(1):39–44.
5. Boyes JH, editor. Bunnell's surgery of the hand. 4th edition. Philadelphia: JB Lippincott; 1964.
6. North ER, Littler JW. Transferring the flexor superficialis tendon: technical considerations in the prevention of proximal interphalangeal joint disability. J Hand Surg Am 1980;5(5):498–501.
7. Brown PW. Reconstructing for pinch in ulnar intrinsic palsy. Orthop Clin N Am 1974;5:323–42.
8. Neviaser RJ, Wilson JN, Gardner MM. Abductor pollicis longus transfer for replacement of first dorsal interosseous. J Hand Surg Am 1980;5(1):53–7.
9. Nemoto K. Restoration of the first dorsal interosseous muscle by transfer of the abductor pollicis longus tendon. Scand J Plast Reconstr Surg Hand Surg 2002;36(4):249–52.
10. Fischer T, Nagy L, Buechler U. Restoration of pinch grip in ulnar nerve paralysis: extensor carpi radialis longus to adductor pollicis and abductor pollicis longus to first dorsal interosseus tendon transfers. J Hand Surg Br 2003;28(1):28–32.
11. Edgerton MT, Brand PW. Restoration of abduction and adduction to the unstable thumb in median and ulnar paralysis. Plast Reconstr Surg 1965;36:150–64.
12. Brand PW. Tendon transfers for median and ulnar nerve paralysis. Orthop Clin North Am 1970;1:447–54.
13. Hirayama T, Atsuta Y, Takemitsu Y. Palmaris longus transfer for replacement of the first dorsal interosseous. J Hand Surg Br 1986;11(1):84–6.
14. De Abreu LB. Early restoration of pinch grip after ulnar nerve repair and tendon transfer. J Hand Surg Br 1989;14:309–14.
15. Graham WC, Riordan D. Sublimis transplant to restore abduction of index finger. Plast Reconstr Surg 1947;2(5):459–62.
16. Nobuta S, Sato K, Kanazawa K, et al. Effects of tendon transfer to restore index finger abduction for severe cubital tunnel syndrome. Ups J Med Sci 2009;114(2):95–9.

Correction of the Claw Hand

Anthony Sapienza, MD[a],*, Steven Green, MD[b]

KEYWORDS

- Intrinsic paralysis • Claw hand • Tendon transfers
- Capsulodesis

Intrinsic paralysis can be the manifestation of a variety of pathologic entities such as stroke, cerebral palsy, Charcot-Marie-Tooth, muscular dystrophy, leprosy, trauma, cervical disease, and compressive and metabolic neuropathies. Patients may present with a spectrum of clinical findings dependent on the cause and severity of the disease. The 3 main problems caused by intrinsic weakness of the fingers are clawing with loss of synchronistic finger flexion, inability to abduct and adduct the digits, and weakness of grip. Smith[1] in 1987 estimated that the intrinsic musculature contributes up to 60% to grip strength. Kozin[2] in 1999 simulated low median or low ulnar nerve lesions in healthy individuals via nerve blocks and determined that the average decrease in grip strength was 38% after ulnar nerve block and 32% after median nerve block. Clawing is defined as hyperextension of the metacarpophalangeal (MCP) joints and flexion of the interphalangeal (IP) joints (**Figs. 1** and **2**). The Zancolli classification[3] distinguishes between intrinsic paralysis with and without claws. Intrinsic paralysis without claw can occur when the extrinsic muscles are also paralyzed (as seen in high ulnar nerve palsy involving the flexor digitorum profundus (FDP) to the ring and small fingers) or conservation of the activity of the corresponding finger lumbrical (as seen with the median nerve innervated lumbricals of the index and middle fingers in ulnar nerve palsy). There may be other rarer causes, which prevent hyperextension of the MCP joint: congenital shortness of the volar plate, spasticity or contracture of the intrinsic muscles, intrinsic tendon adhesions at the level of the MCP joint, fascial or skin contractures (eg, burns, scarring, Dupuytren disease). The observation of such rare cases had initially led Zancolli to propose his capsulodesis in the treatment of claw deformity.[4]

Patients may initially present with subtle findings such as weakness of pinch or an abducted posture of the small finger. A palsied first dorsal interosseous muscle affects thumb–index finger pinch, and stabilization of the index finger is usually accomplished by bracing it against the middle finger. On some occasions a patient requires surgery to restore index finger abduction, especially when considering transfers to restore thumb-index pinch (see Lee and Wisser elsewhere in this issue for further exploration of this topic). Pinch may also be affected by weakness of the adductor pollicis. In these cases, acute flexion of the IP joint via the flexor pollicis longus allows the extensor pollicis longus to exert an adduction moment on the thumb because the IP extensor action is blocked (Froment sign,[5] **Fig. 3**). The thumb MCP joint may hyperextend during pinch (Jeanne sign[6]) if there is thumb volar plate laxity and both heads of the flexor pollicis brevis are paralyzed.

Chronic abduction of the small finger results from the inability of the palsied third palmar interossei to counteract the force of the extensor digiti quinti (EDQ). This extrinsic extensor to the small finger exerts an MCP joint extension force

The authors have nothing to disclose.

[a] Hand Surgery Division, Department of Orthopedics, Bellevue Hospital Center, NYU Hospital for Joint Diseases, 301 East 17th Street, New York, NY 10003, USA
[b] 2 East 88th Street, New York, NY 10128, USA
* Corresponding author.
E-mail address: anthony.sapienza@nyumc.org

Hand Clin 28 (2012) 53–66
doi:10.1016/j.hcl.2011.09.009

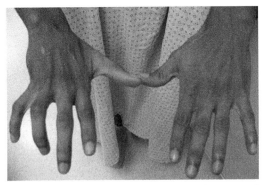

Fig. 1. Clawing of right ring and small fingers with noted intrinsic muscle and hypothenar atrophy.

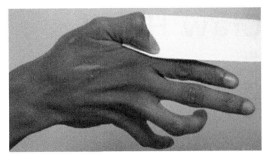

Fig. 3. Froment's sign.

as well as produces small finger abduction (Wartenberg sign,[7] **Fig. 4**) because of its ulnar insertion to the abductor digiti quinti at the level of the proximal phalanx.

The typical finger clawing appearance of the hand is caused by weakness of the intrinsics and unopposed pull of the extrinsic extensors and flexors, because the function of the intrinsic musculature is to flex the MCP joints and extend the IP joints. In ulnar nerve paralysis this situation typically affects the ring and small finger clawing deformity (Duchenne sign,[8] see **Fig. 2**) and weakness of the flexion of the middle and index MCP joints. Clawing of the index and middle fingers does not occur in cases of ulnar nerve dysfunction because their lumbricals are innervated by the median nerve. Complete ulnar nerve palsy may result in clawing of only the small finger because the ring finger lumbrical has dual innervation in up to 50% of the population.[1] The level of peripheral nerve dysfunction determines the clinical presentation and may guide treatment options. For example, a high ulnar nerve palsy (above the motor branches to the flexor carpi ulnaris and ring and small finger FDP muscles) involves paralysis of the flexor digitorum profundi to the ring and small finger and thus produces less clawing than does a low ulnar nerve palsy.

Differences in the claw presentation can also be attributed to anomalous innervations of the muscles of the hand and forearm[9] as well as a variety of pathologic causes. The clinical appearance of the claw and its severity are also dependent on the laxity of the MCP joints. Although IP joint extension is primarily via the intrinsic musculature, the extrinsic extensors can normally extend the IP joints provided that the MCPs do not hyperextend and the extensor mechanism at the proximal interphalangeal (PIP) joint has not become stretched. If the MCP joint is hyperextended then the extrinsic musculature has approached its limit of excursion at this joint and forces cannot be transmitted distally through the central slip to extend the PIP joint. If MCP joint hyperextension is prevented, the extrinsic extensors can produce IP extension as long as joint contractures and stretching of the PIP extensor mechanism have not ensued (Bouvier test,[10] **Fig. 5**).

In the absence of intrinsic function, MCP flexion occurs only after IP joint flexion, rather than simultaneously, inhibiting the grasp of large objects (**Fig. 6**).

This loss of synchronistic flexion of the MCP and IP joints makes it difficult for the patient to

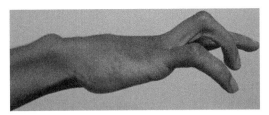

Fig. 2. Clawing of ring and small finger with MCP joint hyperextension and IP joint flexion.

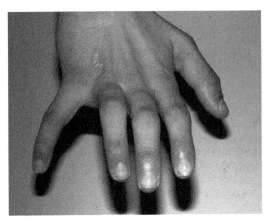

Fig. 4. Wartenberg's sign.

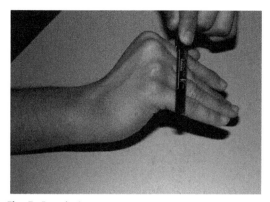

Fig. 5. Bouvier's test.

accommodate objects for grasp and results in a rolling or curling motion of the digits into flexion (**Fig. 7**).

The clawed fingers grasp large objects only with the tips and at the metacarpal heads. Brand[11] has estimated that this situation results in a 90% reduction in the contact area and therefore a significant increase in pressure localization. In attempting to improve finger extension, the wrist may assume a flexed position (André-Thomas[12] sign, **Fig. 8**).

CLINICAL EVALUATION

When evaluating a patient who presents with intrinsic weakness several questions need to be addressed to guide what, if any, treatment is warranted. A lack of patient commitment and compliance results in unfavorable outcomes regardless of the intervention. Along with identifying the motor deficits (claw, thumb-index pinch, Wartenberg sign, and Froment sign) the examiner should also determine the active and passive motion of the

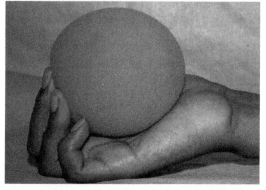

Fig. 6. Intrinsic paralysis results in failure to accommodate around large objects.

digits and their sensibility. Is there adequate sensibility? The outcomes of surgery can be improved if sensibility can be restored. Can the claw deformity be passively corrected? Joint stiffness and contractures need to be addressed before considering any tendon transfer procedures. If the MCP joints are held in flexion, can the patient actively extend the IP joints? If the MCP joints are taken out of hyperextension, the extrinsic extensors are then allowed to exert their force through the central slip to extend the IP joints (Bouvier test). Depending on the chronicity of the claw and the degree of MCP joint hyperextension, the extensor mechanism may have stretched out with time. In this situation, the MCP joints may need to be flexed beyond neutral to produce enough tension on the extensor mechanism to allow it to pull through. The degree of MCP joint flexion necessary to allow for IP extension can guide the examiner's treatment options (**Fig. 9**).

If the patient is able to extend the IP joints with MCP joint flexion up to about 40°, then the Bouvier test is considered positive, and a lumbrical bar splint may be all that is necessary to improve the patient's function (see the article by Seu and Milano elsewhere in this issue for further exploration of this topic). If the MCP joints need to be flexed beyond 40°, then significant stretching of the PIP extensor mechanism has ensued and dynamic tendon transfers to the lateral bands is indicated to improve the clawing.

Does the patient complain of reduced grip strength? If so, then dynamic tendon transfers are the only intervention that can correct this problem. If tendon transfer procedures are being considered, then what are the expendable and appropriate motor donors and what is the quality of the soft tissues along the path of the tendon transfer? In 1988, Brand[13] discussed how the mechanical properties of the peritendinous scar can affect the success of a tendon transfer. If the condition of the soft tissues is poor then delay of surgical intervention until the soft tissues mature or placement of silicon tendon rods to create a smooth gliding bed for the tendon transfer can be considered. In 1919, Steindler[14] advocated delaying tendon transfer surgery until edema is resolved, joints are supple, and scars are soft.

Is there a changing neurologic condition? If the patient's neurologic condition is worsening, then supportive management (stretching or splinting) may be all that is warranted until there has been some stasis of the disease. Likewise, if the patient's neurologic condition is improving then stretching to keep the joints supple and splinting to prevent MCP joint hyperextension may be all that is necessary until intrinsic function returns.

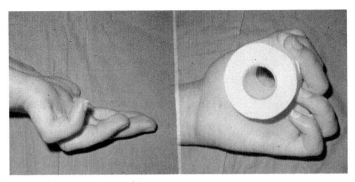

Fig. 7. Rolling and curling of digits to grasp objects.

The motor end plates die off by around 18 months, so even in the presence of an improving neurologic condition, the likelihood that the intrinsics will be reinnervated in a timely fashion must be determined.

SURGICAL TREATMENT OPTIONS

Surgical treatment of a claw hand can involve either static or dynamic procedures. The appropriate choice of procedure should take into account the patient's complaints, goals, and ability to comply with a rehabilitation program. Static procedures have the advantage of being simple and do not require significant postoperative therapy. The disadvantage of a static procedure is that it cannot correct weakness. Static procedures are designed to prevent MCP joint hyperextension or flex the MCP joint so that the IP joints can be extended and are therefore indicated only if the Bouvier test is positive. These procedures include MCP joint arthrodesis, bone block,[15,16] tenodeses, and volar plate capsulodesis. MCP joint arthrodesis of the fingers is rarely performed to prevent clawing because there are other static procedures that can inhibit hyperextension and still permit joint flexion.

Capsulodesis

In the original Zancolli capsulodesis[4] procedure, the volar capsule of the MCP joint is approached through a longitudinal incision centered over the A1 pulley of each involved digit. We recommend using a transverse incision to improve visualization when more than 1 finger requires treatment. The A1 pulley is incised (like a trigger finger release) and the flexor tendons reflected laterally to expose the origin of the volar plate on the metacarpal neck (**Fig. 10**).

In Zancolli's original description the volar plate is then sharply incised and advanced proximally in a "vest over pants" imbrication technique. Late stretching of the capsulodesis and recurrence of MCP joint hyperextension led to several modifications of the procedure. A more reliable technique involves detaching the volar plate off the metacarpal neck and advancing it proximally. The volar plate is sharply released from its origin

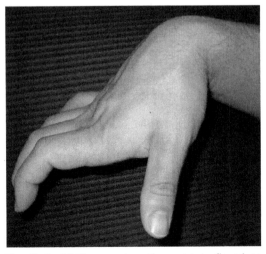

Fig. 8. André-Thomas sign: the wrist is flexed to increase tension on the extrinsics and improve finger extension.

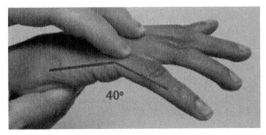

Fig. 9. Bouvier's test.

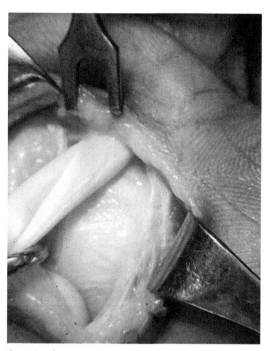

Fig. 10. Flexor tendons reflected laterally, exposing the volar plate.

using a transverse incision at its most proximal border followed by longitudinal incisions extending distally along the radial and ulnar borders of the metacarpal neck, which releases the accessory collateral ligament attachments. Proximal tension with a forceps on this U-shaped flap should induce MCP joint flexion (**Fig. 11**).

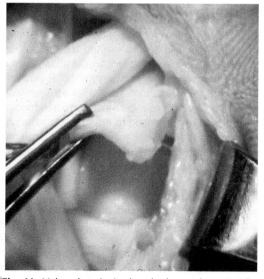

Fig. 11. Volar plate incised and advanced proximally.

The MCP joint is then flexed down to at least the flexion necessary to enable IP joint extension (determined preoperatively by the Bouvier test). In Zancolli's own modification of the procedure[17] the volar plate is then advanced proximally and sutured under tension to the surrounding periosteum. We recommend a modification to this procedure by using a suture anchor to advance the volar plate proximally and reattach it to the metacarpal shaft. The MCP joint can then be flexed to the appropriate degree as determined preoperatively by the Bouvier test and pinned in place using a K-wire. The volar plate can then be advanced under as much tension as possible, giving the surgeon more confidence that the capsulodesis is not too tight or too loose. We also recommend sharply scoring the metacarpal neck to create a bleeding bony bed to facilitate volar plate reattachment. This step would be difficult in the original procedure because of the necessity to conserve as much periosteum as possible. Once the volar plate is secured with a suture anchor, the K-wire can be removed to allow for MCP joint flexion and minimize stiffness. The capsulodesis should be protected with a dorsal blocking splint, which prevents the terminal 30° MCP joint extension for 6 weeks. MCP joints are permitted to flex and IP joints mobilized for the first 6 weeks, followed by 6 weeks of splinting only to prevent inadvertent sudden hyperextension of the MCP joints.

Tenodeses

Several tenodeses have been described that either prevent MCP joint hyperextension or produce PIP joint extension as the MCP joint extension occurs. Tenodeses that only prevent MCP joint hyperextension require tendon grafts and have not shown an advantage over capsulodesis. If the proximal portion of the tenodesis is attached at the wrist level, then finger motion is affected by wrist position. There are several pearls when inserting a tenodesis or tendon transfer into the lateral bands. When performing a midaxial incision along the proximal phalanx, use blunt retractors to keep the neurovascular bundle safely volar. Handle the lateral bands gently to minimize adhesions, which may restrict excursion of the extensor mechanism.

Riordan static tenodesis
The tenodesis of Riordan[18] is a hand-based tenodesis that uses the extensor carpi ulnaris (ECU) and extensor carpi radialis longus (ECRL) tendons, in which only a strip of each tendon is removed and its distal insertion is preserved. The width of each donor tendon is split in half and the split is carried proximally, preferably to the musculotendinous junction. The graft is then reflected in a distal

direction and divided into 2 tails, preserving its distal attachment on the base of the metacarpals (**Fig. 12**). Each tail is then tunneled through the interosseous space and lumbrical canal to reach the radial side of the corresponding finger. The MCP joints are then flexed to the appropriate position (determined preoperatively by the Bouvier test) and the grafts are sutured to the intrinsic lateral band. A period of postoperative splinting is necessary for 4 weeks, maintaining the MCP joints flexed. The IP joints are left free to allow immediate mobilization to prevent stiffness and tendon adhesions.

Fowler's dynamic tenodesis

Fowler[19,20] described a wrist-based tenodesis that weaved a 4-tailed tendon graft through the extensor retinaculum. Each tail of the graft is then passed deep to the transverse metacarpal ligament and attached to the lateral band (**Fig. 13**). The dynamic concept of the tenodesis was that with wrist flexion the graft would tension and because it was passed volar to the transverse metacarpal ligament the tension would produce MCP hyperextension joint flexion and IP joint extension. The tenodesis did not gain widespread favor because

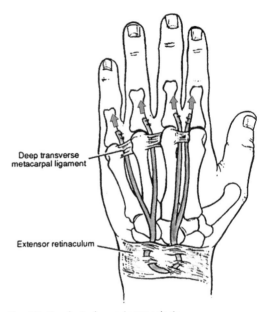

Fig. 13. Fowler's dynamic tenodesis.

it added a level of complexity in correcting a claw deformity without a significant improvement over the simpler capsulodesis procedure. This tenodesis does not improve grip strength because it does not add a motor unit for finger flexion and it does not use synergistic wrist extension during grip activities.

Srinivasan tenodesis

Srinivasan[21] described "the extensor diversion graft operation" for correcting claw deformity and reducing the disability of the intrinsic minus fingers seen in leprosy. The procedure was designed to rebalance the extrinsic extensor dominance at the MCP joint to improve hyperextension and to allow the PIP joints to remain moderately extended when the extrinsic flexors exerted their action on the fingers. Conceptually, this would allow a more synchronous grasp by allowing the MCP joints to flex with the IP joints instead of after as seen with intrinsic palsy. The procedure inserted a free tendon graft, which was attached to the extrinsic extensor just proximal to the MCP joint, passed volar to the transverse metacarpal ligament, and distally attached to the lateral bands. The surgery had to be performed under local anesthetic to set the tension on the graft. One or 2 test stitches were inserted and the patient was asked to extend the finger. If the claw deformity was undercorrected then the finger went into hyperextension at the MCP joint and flexion at the IP joint. If the deformity was overcorrected then the finger assumed an intrinsic-plus position, with deficient flexion at the

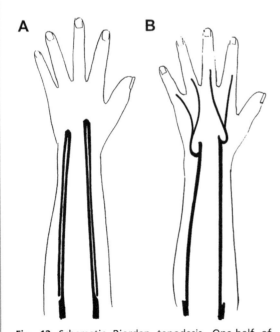

Fig. 12. Schematic Riordan tenodesis. One-half of ECRL and one-half of ECU are used (*A*) and split into a total of 4 tails. Each tail is then routed volar to the deep transverse metacarpal ligament and attached to the lateral band (*B*). (*Reprinted from* Riordan DC. Tendon transplantations in median and ulnar-nerve paralysis. J Bone Joint Surg Am 1953;35:317; with permission.)

MCP joint and full extension at the IP joint. Although the concept of rebalancing the extensor apparatus was novel, and most cases did have a correction of their claw deformity, the investigator noted that it was not possible to predict the functional effect of the operation on the intrinsic minus hand.

Smith sling tenodesis

Smith[22] described a sling tenodesis in which a graft was passed around the deep transverse metacarpal ligament and sutured to the lateral bands of adjacent fingers. The lateral bands are approached through midaxial incisions on the opposing sides of the ring and small or middle and index fingers. A tendon graft is passed proximally through one of the midaxial incisions and dorsal to the deep transverse metacarpal ligament. A curved hemostat is then placed in the other digital incision to retrieve the graft so that it loops around volar to the deep transverse metacarpal ligament. The graft is sutured into one of the lateral bands. The MCP joints are flexed to 30°, whereas the IP joints are extended and the graft is secured to the other lateral band while under tension (**Fig. 14**). This tenodesis produced PIP joint extension as MCP joint extension occurred but did not have a significant impact on synchronous finger flexion and did not augment grip strength.

Dynamic Transfers

Dynamic tendon transfers involve transferring functional muscle-tendon units to restore another by transferring the working unit to a new location. The transfer should involve sacrificing an expendable muscle-tendon unit (eg, 1 wrist extensor donor, extensor carpi radialis brevis [ECRB]; whereas 2 remain, ECRL and ECU) so that hand function remains balanced. Dynamic procedures have the disadvantage of being more complex than static procedures. The advantages of dynamic procedures involve correction of the claw deformity, improving grip strength, restoration of power pinch (see the article by Lee and Wisser elsewhere in this issue for further exploration of this topic), and restoring the synchronistic flexion of the fingers. There have been 2 proposed tendon transfer routes. The volar route involves passing the tendon transfer through the carpal canal and volar to the deep transverse metacarpal ligaments. This technique has been described by Brand[23–25] using a wrist extensor and Bunnell[26] using a flexor digitorum superficialis (FDS). Brand also described his transfer via a dorsal route that places the tendon transfer though the intermetacarpal spaces, then volar to the deep transverse metacarpal ligaments and through the lumbrical canals.

There have been 4 described tendon insertion sites (**Fig. 15**). Brand and Bunnell attached the transferred tendon to the lateral band of the extensor apparatus. Zancolli lassoed his tendon transfer around the A1 pulley, and Omer[27] modified the procedure to loop around the A2 pulley. Burkhalter and Strait[28] fixed the transferred tendon to the proximal phalanx via bone tunnels (**Fig. 16**).

In deciding which insertion site to use the surgeon needs to revisit the Bouvier test. If the

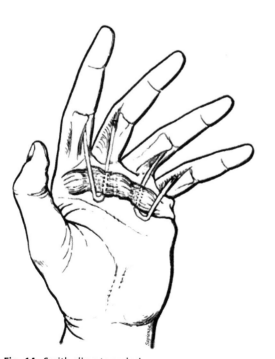

Fig. 14. Smith sling tenodesis.

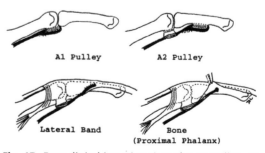

Al Pulley A2 Pulley

Lateral Band Bone
(Proximal Phalanx)

Fig. 15. Four digital insertion sites: the A1 pulley, A2 pulley, lateral band, and bone insertion. (*Reprinted from* Donald HL, Rodriguez JA. Tendon transfers for restoring hand intrinsic muscle function: a biomechanical study. J Hand Surg Am 1999;24(3):609–13; with permission.)

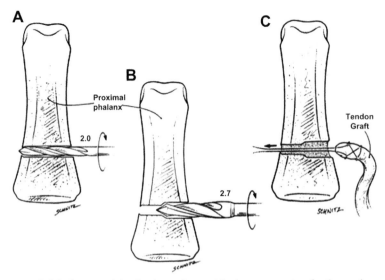

Fig. 16. (*A–C*) 2.0-mm drill hole is used for both cortices, with the near cortex further enlarged with a 2.7-mm drill. (*Reprinted from* Hastings H. Ulnar nerve paralysis. In: Strickland JW, Graham TJ, editors. Master techniques in orthopaedic surgery: the hand. 2nd edition. Philadelphia: Lippincott Williams & Wilkins; 2005. p. 224; with permission.)

Bouvier test is positive then by definition the extensor mechanism is competent to extend the IP joints and the surgeon can consider inserting the tendon transfer into the pulleys of the tendon sheath or directly into the bone of the proximal phalanx. The advantage of these insertion sites is that it is easier to set the tension of the transfer. The usefulness of the bone tunnel insertion site can also be recognized because it has the advantage of a strong bone-tendon interface. If the Bouvier test is negative, then IP joint extension can be accomplished only if the tendon is transferred into the lateral bands.

FDS Transfers

Zancolli lasso
The Zancolli[17] lasso procedure creates a functionally dynamic tenodesis in which each FDS is divided at its insertion on the middle phalanx, looped around its corresponding A1 pulley, and sutured back onto itself to provide flexion of the MCP joints (**Fig. 17**). By definition this is a dynamic transfer, but because it involves rerouting the insertion of a finger flexor, no change in grip strength occurs.[29] This procedure is good for diffuse paralysis or if limited donor tendons are available. The procedure improves the appearance and function of a claw hand only if the Bouvier test is positive. A modification of the Zancolli lasso uses only one-half of the FDS tendon of the middle finger.[30] Omer[27] also modified the procedure to loop the tendon around the A2 pulley. The Zancolli lasso

has the potential of inhibiting FDP gliding because of the increased bulk within the sheath because the FDS tendon is folded back on itself at the level of the Camper chiasm. Another pitfall is that some patients have significant joint laxity and have hyperextensible PIP joints. In these individuals, if the FDS tendon is released at its distal insertion on the middle phalanx then the patient may develop a swan-neck deformity from the unopposed pull of the extrinsic extensors. In these individuals leaving a stump of the FDS at the level of the PIP joint allows it to scar down to the sheath and creates a tether to minimize hyperextension, or the surgeon can suture the stump directly to the sheath to ensure its tethering action.

Stiles-Bunnell transfer
Stiles in 1922[31] was the first author to describe a tendon transfer to the lateral bands to restore intrinsic function. Bunnell modified the technique by transferring all the FDS tendons to the lateral bands of both sides of each clawed digit.[26,32] He found that this transfer was too powerful and caused swan-neck deformities. Littler[33] further modified the technique to use 1 FDS tendon to motor 2 to 4 digits. Midaxial incisions on the radial border of each digit are used to expose the lateral band and flexor sheath. A window in the A3 pulley is used to divide the middle or ring FDS tendon distally. The tendon is then retrieved through a midpalmar incision, split longitudinally into 2 to 4 tails, and each tail is passed through the lumbrical canal volar to the deep metacarpal ligament

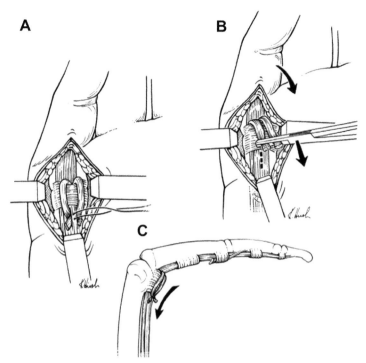

Fig. 17. The Zancolli lasso procedure: the FDS tendon is released from its insertion (*B*) and sutured back to itself over the A1 pulley (*A, C*). (*Reprinted from* Tse R, Hentz VR, Yao J. Late reconstruction for ulnar nerve palsy. Hand Clin 2007:23(3):383; with permission.)

and attached to the lateral bands (**Figs. 18** and **19**). A strong muscle that was previously the prime flexor of the PIP joint now becomes the prime extensor of that same joint and leaves the FDP as the only digital flexor. The sublimus and profundus no longer act synergistically, and reeducation for them to act reciprocally can be difficult.

Tension on the graft is set by using 50% of the available excursion with the wrist neutral, the MCP joints flexed to 60°, and IP joints extended. After transfer into the lateral bands, the wrist is splinted in neutral with MCP joints flexed to 60° and IP joints extended for 1 month. If the Bouvier test is positive then the tendon can be sutured into either the A2 pulley[34] or inserted into a bone tunnel on the radial aspect of the proximal phalanx and tied over a button.[28] If the transfer is into the proximal phalanx or A2 pulley then the IP joints are allowed to immediately mobilize, whereas the wrist and MCP joints remain splinted

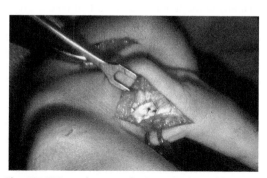

Fig. 18. Middle FDS split into 2 tails and passed down the lumbrical canals of ring and small fingers.

Fig. 19. FDS tendon transfer into the lateral bands.

for 1 month. Brand[23] noted that when performing the FDS tendon transfer the residual stump had scarred down to the sheath in a sort of bowstring across the PIP joint, preventing extension. On excising the bowstring, full joint extension could be obtained. Based on these findings Brand recommended sectioning the FDS tendon exactly at its insertion. A swan-neck deformity can be a complication of this procedure, especially if the patient has hyperlax joints. To minimize this deformity in individuals with significant joint laxity we recommend not sectioning the FDS tendon at its distal most insertion, but instead leaving a stump that can scar down to the surrounding sheath and form a volar tether.

Wrist motor transfers

Using a wrist extensor or flexor can correct claw deformity and increase grip strength. Whenever a wrist motor is used it must be prolonged with a free tendon graft (palmaris longus, plantaris, toe extensor, fascia lata) to achieve digital insertion. Brand suggested performing transfers to all digits because although the median-innervated lumbricals can prevent a claw deformity, they may not have the strength to produce strong MCP joint flexion when resistance is encountered.

Brand ECRB or ECRL transfer

Littler[33] initially described and Brand[23] popularized the procedure that involved a dorsal-based transfer (the so-called Brand I) for the treatment of the paralytic claw hand. The procedure routed the ECRB prolonged with a 4-tailed graft through the intermetacarpal spaces, then volar to the deep transverse metacarpal ligaments, and attached to the lateral bands (**Fig. 20**). We recommend this transfer because it uses the synergistic action of wrist extension, MCP joint flexion, and IP joint extension. In addition to improving claw deformity and synchronistic finger flexion, it improves grip strength by transferring a strong wrist extensor to finger flexor and leaving balanced wrist extension via the ECRL and ECU. Like any of the tendon transfers that take a single motor and split it to empower 4 digits, it can be difficult to obtain an even distribution of force to the recipient digits. For this reason the technical ease of setting the tension to just 2 recipient digits can be considered (eg, a low ulnar palsy in which only the ring and small finger show clawing).

The ECRB tendon is divided at the base of the third metacarpal and mobilized while maintaining its position under the wrist retinaculum. A plantaris or toe extensor tendon graft (the palmaris longus is often too short) is woven through a slit 1 cm from the end of the ECRB secured to the ECRB using

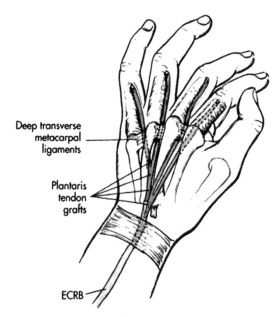

Deep transverse metacarpal ligaments

Plantaris tendon grafts

ECRB

Fig. 20. Brand I transfer.

an interweave suture. This procedure creates a 2-tailed graft that can then be further split longitudinally to create 4 tails. Radial midaxial incisions and dorsal metacarpal incisions are created to allow passage of the tails of the tendon graft from the dorsal wrist, through the lumbrical canals to lie volar to the deep transverse metacarpal ligament (**Figs. 21** and **22**).

Depending on the results of the Bouvier test, the tails can then be inserted into the flexor sheath, proximal phalanx (**Fig. 23**), or laterals bands as discussed earlier.

Tensioning of the transfer is obtained using 50% of the available excursion and inserting the transfer with the wrist held in 30° of extension and the MCP joints in 45° of flexion. If transferring to the lateral bands, the IP joints should also be held in

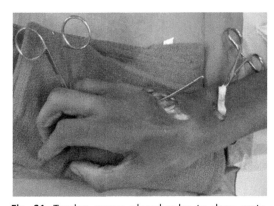

Fig. 21. Tendon passer placed volar to deep metacarpal ligament.

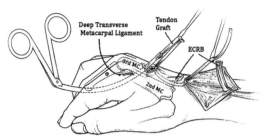

Fig. 22. Dorsal tendon graft routed volar to deep transverse metacarpal ligament.

extension. Proper tensioning of the transfer can be assessed with the wrist held in neutral and noting the MCP joints resting with a flexion attitude of 75°.

Brand[24] in 1961 described a volar-based transfer (Brand II) that routed the prolonged ECRL around the radial side of the wrist by tunneling it deep to the brachioradialis, then through the carpal tunnel, and inserting into each digit as described for the Brand I transfer. The rationale for this modification was to overcome the reeducation component of the Brand I transfer and minimize adhesions that often occurred where the tendon graft perforated the interosseous membrane in the dorsal-based

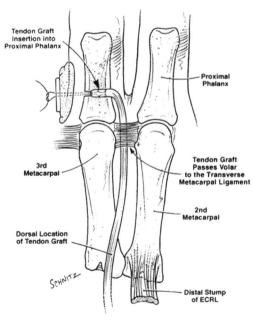

Fig. 23. Tendon graft seated into bone tunnel in proximal phalanx and tied over a button. (*Reprinted from* Hastings H. Ulnar nerve paralysis. In: Strickland JW, Graham TJ, editors. Master techniques in orthopaedic surgery: the hand. 2nd edition. Philadelphia: Lippincott Williams & Wilkins; 2005. p. 224; with permission.)

transfer.[24,35] Brand's patient population was mostly patients with ulnar and median nerve palsy caused by leprosy. We recommend caution when using this transfer, especially in patients who do not have a median nerve palsy, because of the risk of iatrogenic injury when passing the grafts or by increasing the contents of the carpal canal.[1]

Riordan flexor carpi radialis (FCR) transfer

Patients with long-standing claw deformity often have a compensatory flexed posture of the wrist in attempting finger extension (see **Fig. 8**). Riordan[20] described detaching the FCR from its insertion, transferring it to the dorsal side of the forearm, prolonging it with tendon grafts, and then continuing its insertion in a similar fashion to the Brand I transfer described earlier. This transfer overcame the compensatory wrist hyperflexion deformity by rerouting the wrist flexor dorsally. Alternatively, the FCR can be left on the volar side of the forearm, with the prolonged tails routed through the carpal tunnel dorsal to the median nerve and flexor tendons and inserted in a similar fashion to the Brand II transfer described earlier. Like the Brand II transfer, there is the potential risk of median nerve dysfunction.

Palmaris longus transfer

Antia[36] described the benefits of using the palmaris longus as the motor donor, prolonged with tendon grafts, routed through the carpal tunnel, and inserted in a similar fashion to the Brand II transfer. The main function of the palmaris longus is to help cup the hand, and it has a negligible contribution to wrist flexion. It is present in 75% to 80% of the population.[37] It has the mechanical advantage of a direct line of pull. Reeducation of the palmaris transfer after surgery is easy because it contracts whenever the thumb is opposed to the extended digits. Taylor[38] in 2004 compared the clinical outcome of the palmaris longus 4-tailed tendon transfer with the extensor to flexor 4-tailed transfer (Brand II) to correct intrinsic paralysis of the hand in leprosy. After an average follow-up of 33 months the study found there was no statistically significant difference between the 2 groups in terms of active extension lag at the PIP joint, technical outcome, and patient satisfaction. The palmaris longus falls short of providing the combined strength of the intrinsic muscles of the hand.[35] Although it does not provide a significant improvement in grip strength it can diminish clawed appearance of 1 or 2 digits.

Fowler extensor indicis proprius: EDQ transfer

Fowler, in a 1946 personal communication at Valley Forge Hospital as described by Riordan,[18,20] split the extensor indicis proprius (EIP) and EDQ into 2 tails each and passed the tails volar to the transverse metacarpal ligaments through the lumbrical canals and inserted into the lateral bands of each digit. In an isolated ulnar nerve palsy, Riordan[20] modified the procedure to split the EIP into 2 tails and transfer it to the ring and small finger lateral bands only. In a combined median and ulnar nerve palsy, Riordan added a tendon graft to the EIP to create a 4-tailed graft and transfer it to the lateral bands of each digit. Like the other dynamic procedures, the tendon transfer can also be inserted into the proximal phalanx or flexor sheath depending on the Bouvier test. A pearl to the procedure is that the tendons should be harvested with a portion of the extensor hood to provide enough length for reinsertion. Careful closure of the extensor hood is necessary to prevent MCP joint extensor lag and extensor tendon subluxation. The disadvantage of these transfers is that they lack the strength to significantly affect grip, and because they are antagonists to digital flexion, reeducation may also be difficult.

Correction of Wartenberg Sign

Several anatomic studies have noted significant variation in the extensor apparatus to the small finger involving the extensor digitorum communis (EDC), junctura, and EDQ.[39–41] The most frequent pattern of the extensor tendons to the small finger are an absent EDC and a double EDQ with a double insertion[39]; another study reported a similar EDQ pattern, although the EDC to the small finger was present 70% of the time.[40] Blacker and colleagues[41] reported that the ulnar slip of the duplicated EDQ inserted into the ulnar side of the extensor hood at its attachment to the abductor tubercle on the proximal phalanx. The insertion of the extrinsic extensor ulnar to midline creates an abduction vector at the MCP joint when the joint is in extension. If clawing is not present, small finger abduction deformity can be corrected by release of the ulnar slip of the EDQ at its insertion, passing it beneath the radial slip, and inserting it into the radial collateral ligament or radial extensor hood[42] of the small finger MCP joint (**Fig. 24**). If clawing is present, then the claw and small finger abduction deformities can be corrected by transfer of the ulnar slip of the EDQ volar to the deep metacarpal ligament and inserting it into either a bone tunnel in the proximal phalanx, the flexor sheath, or the radial lateral band (depending on the Bouvier test). If the Bouvier test is negative, then IP joint extension can be improved by an insertion into the lateral band.

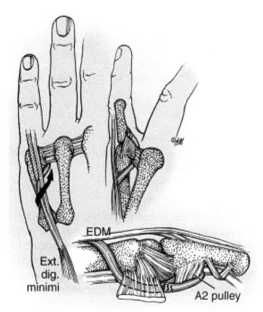

Fig. 24. The ulnar slip of the extensor digiti minimi is passed deep to the transverse metacarpal ligament and inserted into the radial collateral ligament. If the finger is clawed as well as abducted, it can be inserted into the flexor sheath, a bone tunnel in the proximal phalanx, or the lateral band. (*Reprinted from* Davis TR. Median and ulnar nerve palsy. In: Wolfe SW, Hotchkiss RN, Pederson WC, et al, editors. Green's operative hand surgery. 6th edition. Philadelphia: Elsevier Churchill Livingstone; 2011. p. 1131; with permission.)

Chung and colleagues[43] reported on the clinical results of the procedure described by Hoch[44] in which the abducted small finger is corrected by transferring EIP to the distal and radial portion of the extensor hood of the MCP joint of the small finger. The EIP is detached just proximal to the metacarpal head and then the tendinous portion is elongated by splitting it longitudinally except for the most distal 1 cm, where a stay suture is placed to prevent splitting. The split is carried proximally and 1 limb is cut at the musculotendinous junction and turned distally to double the length of the transferred tendon. Multiple sutures are used to reinforce the 1-cm junction of the split tendon limb (**Fig. 25**). The investigators then inserted the transfer to the radial lateral band, but it could also be transferred to the flexor sheath or bone tunnels in the proximal phalanx as described earlier. The transfer is protected in a short-arm splint with the wrist extended 30° and MCP joints in 70° of flexion. After 2 weeks, active motion is then allowed. At a mean follow-up of 23 months all patients had obtained active

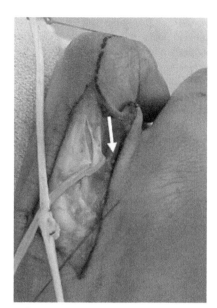

Fig. 25. The EIP tendon is splint longitudinally into 2 parts except for the most distal 1 cm, where a stay suture is placed to prevent splitting. One of the 2 parts is cut at the musculotendinous junction and turned distally to double the length of the transferred tendon. The junction of the split tendon limb is reinforced with multiple sutures. The vector of its pull (*arrow*) is almost parallel to the third palmar interosseous muscle (vessel loop). (*Reprinted from* Chung MS, Baek GH, Oh JH, et al. Extensor indicis proprius transfer for the abducted small finger. J Hand Surg Am 2008;33(3):395; with permission.)

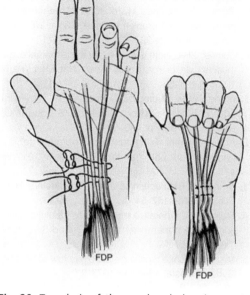

Fig. 26. Tenodesis of the paralyzed ulnar-innervated flexor digitorum profundus tendons of the small and ring finger to the median-innervated middle finger FDP to restore distal IP joint finger flexion. (*Reprinted from* Davis TR. Median and ulnar nerve palsy. In: Wolfe SW, Hotchkiss RN, Pederson WC, et al, editors. Green's operative hand surgery. 6th edition. Philadelphia: Elsevier Churchill Livingstone; 2011. p. 1131; with permission.)

adduction of the small finger without any loss of flexion or extension, and those with a claw deformity showed an improvement with a decrease in PIP joint extension lag.

FLEXOR DIGITORUM PROFUNDUS PALSY

To regain distal interphalangeal joint flexion, a side-to-side transfer of the weakened ulnar-innervated profundi of the ring and small fingers to the median-innervated profundi of the middle finger can be performed through a longitudinal incision along the distal ulnar volar forearm.[27] Tension is set to reproduce the normal digital cascade, and nonabsorbable horizontal mattress sutures are used to secure the profundi together. The index finger profundus can be left free for independent digital motion (**Fig. 26**). The hand is immobilized for 3 weeks with the wrist flexed 20°, MCP joints flexed 45°, and IP joints slightly flexed. Active range of motion is then followed by gentle strengthening with forceful use delayed until 12 weeks after surgery.

REFERENCES

1. Smith RJ. Tendon transfers of the hand and forearm. Boston: Little, Brown; 1987. p. 103–33.
2. Kozin SH, Porter S, Clark P, et al. The contribution of the intrinsic muscles to grip and pinch strength. J Hand Surg Am 1999;24:64–72.
3. Zancolli EA. Tendon transfer after ischemic contracture of the forearm. Classification in relation to intrinsic muscle disorders. Am J Surg 1965;109: 356–60.
4. Zancolli EA. Claw hand caused by paralysis of the intrinsic muscles. A simple surgical procedure for its correction. J Bone Joint Surg Am 1957;39: 1076–80.
5. Froment J. La paralysie de l'adducteur du pouce et le signe de la prehension. Rev Neurol 1914;28:1236.
6. Jeanne M. La deformation du pouce dans la paralysie cubitale. Bull Med Soc Chir 1915;41:703.
7. Wartenberg R. A sign of ulnar palsy. JAMA 1939; 112:1688.
8. Duchenne GB. Physiology of motion. Philadelphia: JB Lippincott; 1949. p. 141–54. [Kaplan EB, Trans].

9. Kaplan ED, Spinner M. Normal and anomalous innervations patterns in the upper extremity. In: Omer GE, Spinner M, editors. Management of peripheral nerve problems. Philadelphia: WB Saunders; 1980. p. 75–99.

10. Bouvier SHV. Note sur une paralysie partielle des muscles de la main. Bull Acad Nat Med (Paris) 1851;18:125–39.

11. Brand PW. In: Hunter JM, Schneider LH, Mackin EJ, editors. Tendon surgery in the hand. St Louis (MO): CV Mosby; 1987. p. 439–53.

12. Andre-Thomas T. Le tonus du poignet dans la paralysie du nerf cunital. Paris Med 1917;25:473.

13. Brand PW. Biomechanics of tendon transfers. Hand Clin 1988;4(2):137–54.

14. Steindler A. Operative treatment of paralytic conditions of the upper extremities. J Orthop Surg 1919;1:608–24.

15. Mikhail IK. Bone block operation for claw hand. Surg Gynecol Obstet 1964;118:1077–9.

16. Howard F, Bunnell S. Surgery of the hand. Philadelphia: JB Lippincott; 1944.

17. Zancolli EA. Intrinsic paralysis of the ulnar nerve–physiopathology of the clawhand. In: Structural and dynamic bases of hand surgery. 2nd edition. Philadelphia: JB Lippincott; 1979. p. 159–206.

18. Riordan DC. Tendon transplantation in median nerve and ulnar nerve paralysis. J Bone Joint Surg Am 1953;35:312–20.

19. As described by Littler JW. Principles of reconstructive surgery of the hand. In: Converse JM, editor, Reconstructive plastic surgery, vol. 4. Philadelphia: Saunders; 1964. p. 1612–95.

20. Riordan DC. Tendon transfers for median, ulnar or radial nerve palsy. Hand 1969;1(1):42–6.

21. Srinivasan H. The extensor diversion graft operation for correction of intrinsic minus fingers in leprosy. J Bone Joint Surg Br 1973;55:58–65.

22. Smith RJ. Metacarpal sling tenodesis. Bull Hosp Joint Dis 1984;44:466–9.

23. Brand PW. Paralytic claw hand. With special reference to paralysis in leprosy and treatment by the sublimis transfer of Stiles and Bunnell. J Bone Joint Surg Br 1958;40B:618–32.

24. Brand PW. Tendon grafting illustrated by a new operation for intrinsic paralysis of the fingers. J Bone Joint Surg Br 1961;43:444–53.

25. Brand PW. Tendon transfers for median and ulnar nerve paralysis. Orthop Clin North Am 1970;1:447–54.

26. Bunnell S. Surgery of the intrinsic muscles of the hand other than those producing opposition of the thumb. J Bone Joint Surg 1942;24:1–31.

27. Omer GE Jr. Ulnar nerve palsy. In: Green DP, editor. Operative hand surgery. 3rd edition. New York: Churchill Livingstone; 1993. p. 1419–66.

28. Burkhalter WE, Strait JL. Metacarpophalangeal flexor replacement for intrinsic-muscle paralysis. J Bone Joint Surg Am 1973;55:1667–76.

29. Hastings H, McCollam SM. Flexor digitorum superficialis lasso tendon transfer in isolated ulnar nerve palsy: a functional evaluation. J Hand Surg 1994;19A:275–80.

30. Narayanakumar TS. Claw-finger correction in leprosy using half of the flexor digitorum superficialis. J Hand Surg Eur Vol 2008;33(4):494–500.

31. Stiles HJ, Forrester-Brown MF. Treatment of injuries of the spinal peripheral nerves. London: Fronde & Hodder-Stoughton; 1922. p. 166.

32. Bunnell S. Surgery of the hand. 2nd edition. Philadelphia: Lippincott; 1948. p. 467–98.

33. Littler JW. Tendon transfers and arthrodesis in combined median and ulnar nerve paralysis. J Bone Joint Surg Am 1949;31:225–34.

34. Brooks AL. A new tendon transfer for the paralytic hand. J Bone Joint Surg Am 1975;57:730.

35. Brandsma JW, Brand PW. Claw-finger correction, Considerations in choice of technique. J Hand Surg Br 1992;17(6):615–21.

36. Antia NH. The palmaris longus motor for lumbrical replacement. Hand 1969;1(2):139–45.

37. White WL. The unique, accessible and useful palmaris tendon. Plast Reconstr Surg Transplant Bull 1960;25:133–41.

38. Taylor NL, Dorai AR, Dick HM, et al. The correction of ulnar claw fingers: a follow-up study comparing the extensor-to-flexor with the palmaris longus 4-tailed tendon transfer in patients with leprosy. J Hand Surg 2004;29A:595–604.

39. Gonzalez MH, Gray T, Ortinau E, et al. The extensor tendons to the little finger: an anatomic study. J Hand Surg Am 1995;20:844–7.

40. von Schroeder HP, Botte MJ. Anatomy of the extensor tendons of the fingers: variations and multiplicity. J Hand Surg Am 1995;20:27–34.

41. Blacker GJ, Lister GD, Kleinert HE. The abducted little finger in low ulnar palsy. J Hand Surg 1976;1(3):190–6.

42. Dellon AL. Extensor digiti minimi tendon transfer to correct abducted small finger in ulnar dysfunction. J Hand Surg Am 1991;16:819–23.

43. Chung MS, Baek GH, Oh JH, et al. Extensor indicis proprius transfer for the abducted small finger. J Hand Surg Am 2008;33:392–7.

44. Hoch J. Correction of post-traumatic adduction insufficiency of the small finger by transposition of the tendon of the extensor indicis muscle. Handchir Mikrochir Plast Chir 1993;25:179–83.

Intrinsic Contractures of the Thumb

Jack Choueka, MD[a,b,*], Susan Craig Scott, MD[b]

KEYWORDS

- Thumb • Contracture • Intrinsic contracture
- Tendon transfer

Stedman's medical dictionary defines contracture in the following way: "Static muscle shortening due to tonic spasm or fibrosis, to loss of muscular balance, to the antagonist being paralysed, or to a loss of motion of the adjacent joint."[1] Thumb function, its prehension and position, its length, and its strength are defining features of the human hand. The loss of this ability due to contracture can be as debilitating and as detrimental to function as complete amputation. An understanding of the normal bony architecture, stabilizing ligaments, and most importantly its powerful and precision-directed supporting musculature is necessary to appreciate the functional loss that occurs as a consequence of intrinsic contracture of the thumb (**Fig. 1**).

The purpose of this article is to describe the many causes of intrinsic contracture, to detail how they are evaluated with an emphasis on how the clinician might distinguish among them, and to delineate the surgical and nonsurgical treatment options currently in use.

ETIOLOGY AND PATHOANATOMY OF INTRINSIC CONTRACTURE OF THE THUMB

An enormous amount of literature deals with the surgical treatment of the thumb deprived of some or all of its intrinsic musculature. Loss of the ability to draw the thumb away from the palm, rotate the tip, and flex to allow strong or precision grasp significantly compromises the thumb's elegant design and its practical use.

Although the prevention of problems is by far the best method of preserving thumb function, the teaching of simple methods of prevention is sometimes neglected. For this reason, the phrase "position of function" or "protected position" was coined in the very earliest days of surgical intervention in the treatment of hand and digit problems. This phrase describes the joint and soft-tissue position in which the hand is immobilized in the postoperative recovery period, or following trauma or illness. The position preserves the soft tissues at maximum length and is the position from which they are most easily mobilized when rehabilitation is begun. With regard to the intrinsic muscles and the small joints of the thumb, this refers to the maintenance of spread of the thumb-index web space. Our understanding of the disability caused by a contracted web regardless of cause preceded our understanding of its surgical and therapeutic correction. Only when numerous articles dealing with tendon transfers to address the adducted malpositioned thumb described the very limited success of these procedures did surgeons realize the importance of first releasing the soft tissue to allow transferred tendons to fully function.[2]

The causes of intrinsic contracture of the thumb are best considered when divided into several broad categories.

Burns

Whether the cause of a burn is heat generated by flame, passage of electrical current, or a caustic chemical, the tissue destruction that results is replaced by fibrous scar in a final common pathway leading to contracture. A traumatic

The authors have nothing to disclose.

[a] Department of Orthopedic Surgery, Maimonides Medical Center, 927 49th Street Brooklyn, NY 11219, USA
[b] Department of Orthopedic Surgery, New York University School of Medicine, 550 First Avenue, NY 10016, USA
* Corresponding author. 927 49th Street, Brooklyn, NY 11219.
E-mail address: jchoueka@gmail.com

Hand Clin 28 (2012) 67–80
doi:10.1016/j.hcl.2011.09.008
0749-0712/12/$ – see front matter © 2012 Elsevier Inc. All rights reserved.

hand.theclinics.com

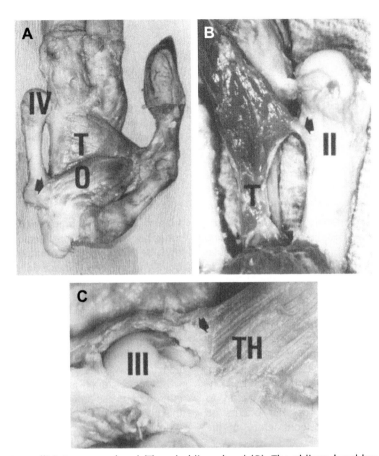

Fig. 1. (*A*) Adductor pollicis transverse head (T) and oblique head (O). The oblique head has an origin (*arrow*) from the base of the ring metacarpal (IV). Muscle of the first ray (*star*) with origins from the trapezium and the thumb metacarpal. (*B*) Transverse head (T) turned ulnarward with an origin from the index metacarpal (II). The structures of the interosseous space have been removed to show the gap between the two metacarpals. (*C*) Transverse head (TH) with its origins from the long metacarpal (III). Muscle fibers originate from the palmar aspect of the metacarpal joint (*arrow*).

syndactyly of the index-thumb web space, a kind of mitten effect, can result from the most severe burns. This complete loss of the ability to abduct renders the thumb useless for opposition. The thenar muscles may be functional, but shortening and contracture will occur if left in this position. Alternatively, the edema and inflammation associated with a burn can be replaced by fibrous scar, also resulting in thenar muscle contracture. Carefully timed debridement, contracture release, coverage, and tendon transfer as needed, along with immobilization in the protected position, comprise the steps leading to the most successful outcome.

Iatrogenic

Immobilization of the thumb ray in a position that ignores the necessity of thumb web spread for even a short period of time can result in adduction contracture. This problem is seen frequently when a practitioner not knowledgable in the concept of small joint protection treats a hand or thumb problem and fails to maintain the span between the index metacarpal and the thumb. When the thumb is immobilized in the plane of the palm, the adductor fibers are foreshortened. Left in this position, the foreshortening will require significant passive stretching to regain full fiber length, and may never be completely reversible.

Ischemic Injury

In the hand the intrinsic muscles of the thumb lie within two separate compartments, the thenar compartment and the adductor compartment. Each compartment is covered with a substantial fascial layer. The intrinsic muscles of the thumb may be subject to ischemic injury by virtue of the anatomic confines in which they are located. Any condition that impairs the blood supply to these muscles or that results in massive hand swelling, such as a crush injury, can result in ischemia, muscle necrosis, and replacement by fibrous contracture, not unlike Volkmann ischemic contracture of the forearm.[3,4] Virtually any cause of massive swelling, be it hemorrhage in an anticoagulated patient, infection, multiple metacarpal fractures, or even the controlled trauma of extensive surgery followed by the placement of the limb in a dependent position, has the potential to result in fibrosis and contracture.

Dupuytren Disease

The fascial contracture of Dupuytren disease can extend to the radial side of the hand, albeit less commonly than its occurrence in the ulnar palm and digits. A variety of patterns of contracture is possible, as the normal fascial alignment in the thumb is both transverse and longitudinal; the longitudinal alignment has the potential to affect both the flexor and abductor surfaces of the thumb.[5] A common pattern is contracture of the proximal commissural ligament, analogous to the transverse component of the palmar fascia frequently seen lying deep when a longitudinal pretendinous cord is excised, and which when affected can result in web-space contracture. Metacarpophalangeal (MP) flexion contracture can occur when the longitudinal band to the thumb is affected, or with involvement of the fascia overlying the abductor brevis. Fascial thickness increases normally the more radially located is the musculature; fascia is thinnest over the flexor pollicis brevis (FPB) and thickest over the abductor pollicis brevis (APB). Contracture of these muscles can result in both abduction and flexion of the thumb.

Congenital

Causes of intrinsic contracture of the thumb occurring at birth are found distributed among the several subcategories of congenital hand differences. Some occur in isolation, but most are one component of a larger syndrome. Virtually all of these conditions result in intrinsic muscle contracture, not as a component of the primary pathology but as a secondary effect of weak or absent balancing musculature, skin and subcutaneous pathology, or primary joint contracture.

Congenital clasped thumb describes a large category of varied congenital thumb deformities; the most easily understood classification was described by McCarroll and subsequently modified by Mih,[6,7] and is based on the clinical evaluation of the deformity. Both investigators

emphasize a clear understanding of the underlying weakness or absence of musculature, and the fixed contracture of skin, ligament, or muscle that makes up the abnormality. Release of structures that are contracted and replacement of structures that are inadequate or absent is necessary. Arthrogryposis multiplex congenita is an example of this group of congenital deformities. A condition of primary static nonprogressive joint contracture, arthrogryposis creates secondary contractures of the adductor muscle as well as the skin and soft tissues of the web space. These conditions, of which Freeman-Sheldon (whistling face) syndrome is another typical example, are inherited as autosomal dominant, though there can be some variation in penetrance.

Contracture of the thumb occurs as a component of other congenital disorders such as syndactyly or Apert syndrome. Apert syndrome, craniosynostosis in conjunction with complex syndactyly, is a genetic mutation that sometimes presents with the thumb encompassed by the syndactylous hand mass. The contracture in this case involves the skin and soft tissues of the web space, the thenar musculature, and the ligaments of the basal joint, and treatment addresses all contracted or absent components.[8]

Among conditions that result in secondary muscle contracture requiring release is congenital dystrophic epidermolysis bullosa, a cutaneous abnormality affecting the structure of skin whereby the various skin laminae separate, blister, and scar secondarily. It is this scarring leads to contracture not only of skin but also of underlying musculature, which results in secondary syndactyly of digits including the thumb.[9] The structural skin defect is the inherited abnormality present at birth; though not a congenital hand difference in the usual sense, its presentation requires release of contracted muscle in addition to the necessary skin replacement and coverage.

Inflammatory

Inflammatory pathologies vary significantly in their thumb involvement, and are well described. Recent advances in the medical treatment of inflammatory diseases have reduced the number of patients requiring surgical intervention. Conditions that could be anticipated such as secondary joint contractures were at one time best treated by prevention. The release of contracted structures, the rerouting of displaced tendons, and the transfer of functioning units to replace those that have ruptured all now take place with diminished frequency.

While all 3 joints of the thumb ray may be involved with intrinsic contracture occurring secondarily, in inflammatory conditions such as rheumatoid arthritis other factors are likely at play in the intrinsic muscle tightening that occurs. There is some evidence that elevated levels of matrix metalloproteinases found in the invasive tenosynovium of rheumatoid arthritis may be responsible for tendon ruptures that occur in this disease which, if left untreated, may result in fibrosis and contracture of muscle.[10]

In addition, significant muscle hypoxia has been demonstrated in rheumatoid arthritis; the resulting fibrosis of hypoxic muscle may also contribute to muscle contracture.[11]

As the joints swell with synovial proliferation and the soft-tissue support deteriorates both from direct involvement and from passive stretch, secondary changes occur. Nalebuff[12] described variations in thumb posture that occur in rheumatoid arthritis, and a short description of these deformities beginning with the most common is warranted. Nalebuff has categorized these changes as types I to IV; later this was broadened to include two additional categories. Type I, a boutonniere deformity, is most commonly seen, followed in frequency by Type III, a swan-neck deformity. In a Type I deformity, MP flexion results from stretching of the dorsal capsule and of the extensor pollicis brevis along with ulnar and volar subluxation of the extensor pollicis longus (EPL) tendon. The EPL tendon becomes a flexor rather than extensor of the MP joint; this result can also be seen with rupture of the EPL tendon at the wrist. With time the deformity becomes a fixed MP flexion contracture with shortening of FPB as well as the volar joint capsule, both of which require release. Underappreciated is the radial abduction of the thumb metacarpal that results from an attempt to compensate for the marked MP joint flexion. Termed an extrinsic minus deformity, the boutonniere of the rheumatoid thumb is most severe when it begins at the MP joint. When it begins at the interphalangeal (IP) joint with hyperextension, the MP deformity tends to be less marked and the contracture less pronounced.

By contrast, metacarpal adduction with contracture can occur in the Type II, III, and IV rheumatoid thumbs. Type III begins with inflammation at the basal joint; loss of support results in radial subluxation or even dislocation of the joint, and in an imbalance of abduction-adduction force in which the adductor commonly wins and becomes contracted. A similar result occurs in a Type IV deformity, though by a different mechanism. Here disease begins on the ulnar side of the MP joint; loss of the ulnar collateral ligament deviates the distal and proximal phalanges of the

thumb radially, and the adductor pulls the metacarpal into the web. Of note is that the basal joint is ordinarily spared. Type II rheumatoid disease involves all 3 joints and results in adduction contracture.

Systemic lupus erythematosus (SLE) is among the inflammatory causes of intrinsic contracture of the thumb; it differs from rheumatoid disease in that joint destruction is not the main component of the disease. Rather, joint swelling followed by support-altering laxity of the ligaments and the volar plate on which joint stability depends are the hallmarks of SLE. In the thumb, early changes can create passively correctable flexion deformity of the MP joint as the EPL tendon subluxates. Left untreated this deformity will progress to a typical Type I deformity with abduction of the thumb metacarpal.[13,14]

Scleroderma or systemic sclerosis is a condition in which fibrosis of the skin and soft tissues leads to significant contracted deformities of the hands, especially the digits. The disease affects internal organs as well, including the lungs, gastrointestinal tract, and the kidneys. Severe joint contracture along with thinning and ulceration of the skin is typical. When the thumb is affected, narrowing of the web space with severe adduction contracture along with loss of ability to oppose the thumb is characteristic.[15–17]

No discussion of intrinsic contracture of the thumb would be complete without mention of basal joint osteoarthritis. In certain patients the basal joint is uniquely vulnerable to degeneration of the articular surfaces; this is followed by radial and dorsal subluxation of the metacarpal base as the metacarpal assumes an increasingly flexed and adducted posture. If adduction contracture is present and is not relieved by the partial or total trapezium resection with which this condition is often treated, formal release of the adductor muscle from its origin may be necessary.

Traumatic

Although trauma to the thumb does not commonly result in contracture, a short review of fractures and lacerations affecting the thumb that can result in contracture is necessary.

Severely comminuted thumb metacarpal fractures can result in shortening and collapse.[18] Despite the fact that intra-articular fractures of the thumb require precise anatomic reduction of the joint, extra-articular fractures are surprisingly well tolerated even with a less than perfect reduction of angulation. Accurate evaluation of these injuries requires a true lateral view of the metacarpal, as a severely flexed metacarpal fracture can create MP joint hyperextension; flexion contracture with or without adduction may result. Secondary adduction contracture may result from shortening of the effective length of the metacarpal.

Also in the category of traumatic causes are secondary effects from high-pressure injection injury. The severity of these injuries may not be recognized initially, as the skin wound is often innocuous in appearance immediately after the injury. Even when recognized and extensively debrided, the final common pathway of inflammation and fibrosis may lead to intrinsic contracture of the extrinsic flexor tendon, the affected joints, and the thenar musculature.[19,20] This result can be attributable to direct injection of the noxious substance into the thenar muscles or from a massive local inflammatory reaction.

Infection

The mechanism by which local infection contributes to intrinsic contracture of the thumb must be separated from the stiffness that can occur as a result of purulent infection of the flexor pollicis longus tendon sheath, or from the secondary effect of improper thumb positioning in immobilization implemented as a component of the treatment of such infection.

Any purulent infection of the thenar space, defined as the volar palmar area between the vertical midpalmar septum and the thumb MP joint, can result in adduction contracture of the thumb.[21] Adequate drainage of the space is a sine qua non of appropriate treatment, along with progressive mobilization once the patient's condition permits.

There are less common are chronic infections of the hand, which may be viral, bacterial, fungal, protozoan, or parasitic in origin. Many of these have cutaneous manifestations whose persistence raises suspicion. Among these are Hansen disease, tuberculosis and the atypical mycobacteria, and sporotrichosis. Cryptococcal infection, histoplasmosis, and candidiasis all can mimic arthritis and can present with swollen joints and an absence of cutaneous manifestations, which would raise suspicion of infectious etiology. Tuberculous arthritis most typically presents in the wrist but can affect any of the small joints of the thumb, and should be suspected whenever drainage persists from a joint despite adequate antibiotic treatment.[22] While this group of chronic infections does not primarily target the thenar muscles, chronic, prolonged inflammation and the sequence of local edema, replaced by fibrosis, represent the final common pathway ending in contracture, even when the infection is eradicated.

Neurogenic

Primary neurologic causes of secondary contracture of the intrinsic muscles of the thumb can be central, spinal, or peripheral. Within the group of central causes lie cerebral palsy (CP), brain injury, and stroke. The spinal group comprises those patients with cord injury. Brachial plexus injuries, both preganglionic and postganglionic, along with loss of peripheral nerve due to laceration or severe compression, make up the third neurogenic cause of intrinsic contracture.

The thenar muscles, as an end organ of the nervous system, have a characteristic response to loss of enervation regardless of cause. This response is reviewed here, followed by a description of characteristic changes associated with central, spinal, or peripheral nerve injury. The agonist/antagonist role is reviewed as it relates to intrinsic contracture in the thumb.

The skeletal muscle fibers of which the thenars are composed react to loss of enervation with atrophy, and a reduction in the size, strength, and weight of the muscle fiber.[23] The longer the motor fiber is without its nerve supply, the less is the fiber able to recover following reenervation. For reasons not completely understood at present, some denervated muscle fibers will progress to fibrotic replacement of the fiber followed by contracture.[24] The antagonist of a denervated muscle plays an even more important role in contracture of neurogenic origin. The antagonist, unopposed now in its activity, will contract, and that sustained contracture over time may become fixed. This fact explains the etiology of contracture in a wide variety of primary neurologic abnormalities. Both the agonist, from fibrous degeneration of the motor fiber following prolonged denervation, and the antagonist, from sustained unopposed firing, result in contracture; the ultimate deformity ordinarily leans toward the motor group with continued innervation.

Cerebral palsy

There are two theories concerning the central nervous system disorder that results in a diagnosis of CP. The first is that this static, nonprogressive disorder results from a hypoxic brain injury in the perinatal period. A second more controversial view holds that the disorder is one of abnormal fetal development.[24,25] Regardless of cause, the end result is weakness of some muscle groups affecting the thumb, commonly the extensor abductor group, with a deficit in voluntary motor control.[25] Thumb flexion and adduction is now weakly opposed or completely unopposed, leading over time to the typical thumb-in-palm deformity along with other upper and lower limb abnormalities. The contracting muscles may be spastic, the treatment of which is described here. However, fibrous contracture, when it occurs, is permanent. It is essential in CP to analyze the deforming elements; the cooperation of a team approach of physician, occupational therapist, parent and, where possible, patient cannot be overemphasized. House and colleagues[26] have clearly elucidated the varied thumb deformities seen; to meet with success, treatment must release contracture, stabilize joints, and rebalance motor function.[27]

Stroke and brain injury

Cerebrovascular accident and brain injury both cause the death of upper motor neurons through hemorrhage, embolus, or thrombus.[28] While these conditions may be accompanied by sensory and cognitive deficits, motor impairment commonly manifests as an initial period of flaccidity followed by the progressive contracture of muscle groups that are spared and whose innervation persists. Persistent contracture is accompanied by fibrosis, which is irreversible.

Spinal cord injury

Injury to the cervical spinal cord results in loss of function of the affected motor unit, comprising the lower motor neuron of the anterior horn cell, the axon of that cell, and the muscle fibers innervated by the cell. The precise pattern of injury depends on the level and the extent of the cord injury. Initial paralysis may be followed by some degree of recovery. Motor units above the level of the injury will be unaffected. Again, unopposed muscles whose function is preserved will dominate. Some balance will be reestablished if recovery occurs, but if imbalance persists, contracture of unopposed muscle groups and fibrous degeneration of affected muscles may occur.

Spinal cord injury differs from upper motor neuron loss in several respects. Initial flaccid paralysis affects all muscle groups below the level of injury. As time passes and edema subsides, cord reflexes below the injury level are activated as the inhibition of upper motor neurons is lost. Severe massive spasticity may occur in response to pain, and muscle tone is increased even in the absence of stimuli.[29] The imbalance of spasticity and flaccidity leads to contracture in association with spinal cord injury.

Peripheral nerve injury

Stretch injury, avulsion of or direct laceration of the components of the brachial plexus, lacerations of peripheral nerves, and even chronic, long-standing peripheral nerve compression can result in muscle contracture affecting the intrinsic muscles of the thumb. Low median nerve palsy or compression of the median nerve left untreated can cause marked atrophy of the thenar muscles, which are the primary abductors of the thumb metacarpal. Contracture of the antagonist of these muscles, the adductor, frequently accompanies thenar atrophy and narrows the web space.

Thenar muscle contracture as a sequela of brachial plexus injury is unusual; when thenar muscles are affected the global nature of these injuries effectively eliminates the agonist antagonist imbalance that causes most neurogenic contracture, and weakness or paresis predominates. However, careful attention to splinting along with excellent trauma care and the evolution of techniques in nerve repair and nerve transfer as surgical solutions have made intrinsic contracture associated with brachial plexus injury rare.

EVALUATION

While highly individualized to the presenting condition, the workup and eventual treatment of a patient with an intrinsic contracture of the thumb must consider the overall function of the patient, ability to use the thumb in relation to the hand, the condition of the rest of the hand and proximal extremity, and expectations of both patient and physician. Thumb contractures rarely present in isolation, and a coordinated plan to address patient function will undoubtedly involve other parts of the hand and even the proximal extremity. Often, repeated examinations are needed before formulating ultimate treatment decisions.

History

The history should begin with determining the cause of the contracture, which will help guide the remaining history and examination. In children, a detailed birth history and other related conditions should be elicited. The duration and progression of the contracture should be noted with particular attention to the effect on thumb and hand function. Pain in the thumb and surrounding areas of the hand should be noted. Previous treatments including use of any splints or assistive devices with emphasis on their effect on the condition should be documented. Patients' perceptions of their functional limitations with specific examples should be discussed, and it is at this time that patients' expectations and wishes are determined. An occupational and social history will help focus patients' needs.

Physical Examination

The examination begins at first sight with attention to how the patient uses the thumb and hand to manipulate his or her environment and perform activities such as filling out patient forms. The presence of any deformities, swelling, and skin integrity should be noted. The quality of the skin is assessed by looking for web-space contractures and skin elasticity (**Fig. 2**).

The resting posture of the thumb will give an indication as to cause and severity. The thumb can be adducted with retroposition with MP and IP extension or assume a flexed posture with carpometacarpal (CMC), MP, and IP flexion, such as in thumb-in-palm deformity.

When examining the thumb a distinction between spasticity and fixed contracture should be made, as this has implications in the selection of proper treatments. Spasticity is defined as an involuntary, velocity-dependent, increase in resistance to the stretch of a muscle, as opposed to a contracture, which offers a fixed resistance to a passive stretch due to either joint stiffness or muscle fibrosis. Spasticity has 5 classic characteristics. (1) Selectivity: depending on the joint involved, there are usually specific muscles that become spastic leading to classic deformities. In the thumb, the adductor pollicis is the most frequently involved in spastic conditions such as CP leading to the typical adducted thumb posture seen. (2) Muscle elasticity whereby increasing stretch increases resistance of the muscle. (3) Present at rest but increased with movement, fatigue, pain, or emotional stress. (4) Enhanced reflexes. (5) The presence of synkinesis, whereby muscles incapable of voluntary movement contract in association with contraction of other muscles.[25] Conversely, fibrous contractures cannot be overcome with passive stretch. The difference is often difficult to determine on physical examination, especially in children, and therefore other methods of evaluation are sometimes needed including motor blockade or electromyography (EMG).

Measurement of the first web-space angle is assessed using goniometers to measure angles, or rulers to measure distances between the thumb and index finger.[30] Soft-tissue and bony landmarks for making these assessments have been described. Because comparison with the contralateral extremity is only useful with unilateral involvement, normal web-space angles have been studied. Using bony landmarks such as the index and thumb metacarpals, 40° to 45° has been considered normal.[31,32] A simple technique that does not require specialized equipment and uses soft-tissue landmarks has been described by Jensen and colleagues.[33] The measurement is made by placing the hand flat on a piece of paper, fully abducting the thumb and adducting the fingers. A pen is used to outline the web space and 3 areas are marked with a dot, including the radial border of the index MP, the ulnar border of the thumb IP, and the deepest portion of the web space. The 3 dots are connected by 2 lines and the angle formed is measured. Jensen and colleagues[33] found the mean angle in normal volunteers to be approximately 100°; they also found that simulating a 30° contracture by placing the volunteers in a blocking splint led to abnormal function, which worsened with simulation of a 60° contracture.

Evaluation should include measurements of thumb opposition by asking the patient to touch the thumb to the little finger and measuring any distance remaining. Passive and active motion at the thumb MP and IP joint should be compared with the contralateral extremity.

Joint stability of the CMC, MP, and IP joints of the thumb requires particular attention. Without joint stability, the usefulness of the thumb as a post is hampered. In addition, if tendon transfers are considered to augment strength, they require stable joints through which the muscles can exert their forces.

Individual muscle testing of the thumb can be challenging, but essential, to determine cause of the contracture and help develop treatment plans. When considering tendon transfers, an assessment of the transferring tendons and their corresponding muscles must confirm their usefulness. In particular, the brachioradialis, flexor carpi radialis, flexor digitorum superficialis, and palmaris longus are often used for transfers to augment thumb function. Through observation and palpation, individual intrinsic function of the thumb can be determined. For example, in thumb contractures in

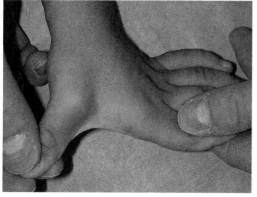

Fig. 2. Child with cerebral palsy, an adduction contracture of the thumb, and a web-space contracture.

patients with CP, the adductor pollicis is nearly always involved with inconsistent involvement of the other intrinsic muscles of the thumb. When the FPB is also involved it causes MP joint flexion, bringing the tip of the thumb toward the little finger; when not involved the thumb and index metacarpals are drawn together without MP flexion.[27,34]

Hand sensibility is assessed by 2-point discrimination, temperature, touch, and stereognosis. Volitional control and hand hygiene are important parameters in assessing in patients with CP and after a stroke, as many believe it corresponds to outcome. Jebsen-Taylor hand function assessments are often used, especially in children; however, recently its validity and responsiveness in measuring hand function has been questioned.[35]

Imaging

Radiographs are needed to assess joint integrity and congruency. Stress views or examination under fluoroscopy may be needed to assess joint stability, particularly at the CMC and MP joints of the thumb. Arthritic changes of the joints may necessitate excision or fusion. Contralateral views are needed when assessing children with contractures, as they may reveal evidence of growth disturbances. Magnetic resonance imaging has limited usefulness in the general workup of thumb contractures.

Motor Blockade

When cocontractions of antagonistic muscles preclude testing for spasticity, motor blocks can be used to make the distinction between a contracture and spasticity of a specific muscle. A variety of pharmacologic agents has been described for motor blocks including lidocaine, diluted alcohol, and phenol.[25] Botulinum toxin injections have the advantage of few side effects and longer-lasting benefits, up to 6 months, providing both a diagnostic and therapeutic intervention.

Neurologic Studies

Nerve conduction studies and EMG may be needed if a neurologic cause is suspected, and to assess the quality of muscles considered for transfer. EMG recordings of specific muscles can help differentiate voluntary capacity from spastic reaction, and dynamic EMG can be used to determine the relative contribution of specific muscle groups such as the adductor when discussing intrinsic thumb contractures.

Hoffer and colleagues[36] used EMG to assess patients with CP and adduction contractures of the thumb. In those with selective control of the adductors only a partial myotomy of the adductor

muscle was performed. By retaining the insertion of the oblique head, these patients retained side pinch. In those that had complete releases, impairment of pinch and grasp sometimes developed.

Videotaping

In children with thumb contractures due to CP the taping of therapy sessions, especially with a therapist who has gained the patient's trust, can prove useful in the assessment of the child's needs.

TREATMENT

A variety of treatment options, both surgical and nonsurgical, are available, with their use customized to individual patient needs. The decision to treat is the first assessment made, as some contractures are so mild that they inhibit no function at all. If the ability to grasp large objects with good strength, muscle balance, and joint stability remains, there is no need to recommend treatment. This aspect is especially true in children, for whom splint compliance is an issue.

Prevention and Nonoperative Management

The prevention of an intrinsic contracture from developing or worsening is paramount. Del Pinal and colleagues[37] evaluated the ability to prevent contractures in a variety of conditions, emphasizing edema management, optimal thumb positioning, splinting, wound management, and stable tissue closure. A variety of static and dynamic splints have been described with various devices such as springs and turnbuckles to maintain proper positioning.[38]

There are two general categories of splinting; those that aim to treat a contracture, spastic, or fibrotic muscle with a continuous stretch, and those that position the thumb to simultaneously improve function and prevent secondary contracture. Splinting for thumb contractures aims at placing an abducting force between the thumb and index metacarpals. Carefully designed splints by experienced therapists using a variety of materials are essential in these cases to avoid complications such as inadvertent stretching of the thumb IP joint, leading to ulnar collateral ligament instability. In general, static splinting and serial casting are preferred over dynamic splinting when attempting to correct web-space contractures. The theoretical basis for this includes reversing the histologic changes that occur in a shortened muscle and decreased sensory input from cutaneous and muscle receptors inhibiting spacticity.[39]

In early burn management, splinting is essential to maintain proper web positioning regardless of surgical intervention. In patients with basal joint arthritis, subluxation of the CMC joint will lead to compensatory adduction contractures of the first metacarpal, and a removable hand-based splint will maintain proper web-space distance and help prevent contractures (**Fig. 3**).[40]

Prevention of iatrogenic contractures caused by inappropriate splinting for injury or fractures is essential. When treating conditions that require thumb immobilization for extended periods such as with scaphoid fractures, intrinsic contractures can be avoided by placing the thumb in a position of function with maintenance of web-space distance. When splinting or casting for conditions that do not require thumb immobilization, care should be taken to allow full motion of the thumb, particularly at the basal joint (**Fig. 4**).

Prevention and recurrence are also essential following surgery. External stabilization with K-wires is commonly used to maintain position and prevent contractures after releases. Following extensive soft-tissue injury or debridement, external splinting may not be possible. In these cases K-wires placed internally as a spring splint has been described.[41] This procedure involves bending a K-wire into one of several configurations such as a "V" or "W" and placing each end through drill holes in the thumb and index metacarpals, where the tension in the K-wire acts as a spring to maintain the proper distance for the web space.

Intrinsic Releases

Releases of contracted muscles are the mainstay of treatment for intrinsic contractures of the thumb. Each muscle unit must be addressed individually to determine the need for release. The adductor pollicis is the most commonly involved, and leads to debilitating loss of thumb function. Release of the adductor can be performed from its origin or its insertion. To avoid unduly weakening thumb

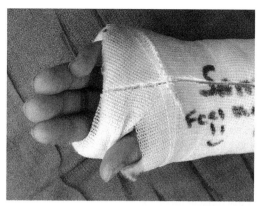

Fig. 4. Arm cast causing adduction contracture of the thumb should be avoided.

adduction, most surgeons advocate the release from its origin on the third metacarpal.[42,43] This action requires an incision along the thenar crease with careful dissection to avoid neurovascular structures. The digital neurovascular bundles and the flexor tendons to the index and long finger are identified and protected. The deep palmar arch and the deep branch of the ulnar nerve are also in the vicinity and at risk for injury. The adductor can be completely released or undergo selective tenotomy of tight tendinous fibers along the muscle distally.[44] Release from its origin allows the adductor to heal in a lengthened position in relation to surrounding structures, preserving some of its function. Release from its insertion, while technically easier and obviating the risks of injury to the neurovascular structures, obliterates the function of the adductor.[43] If releases are performed at the muscle insertions through the first web space, the incisions must be designed to avoid contractures by placing them at 45° to 90° angles to the web.[45]

An exquisite anatomic dissection and anatomic evaluation of the adductor pollicis was performed by Witthaut and Leclercq,[46] who found anatomic variations that help explain surgical failures in some cases. These investigators concluded that to achieve complete release of the adductor, transverse head release must include soft-tissue origins from the fascia of the second interosseous space and osseous origins from the distal third of the index metacarpal reaching as far distally as the MP joint. The oblique head required release from the bases of the 3 middle digits, the capitate, and trapezoid.

When adductor release alone does not allow proper thumb positioning, the other thumb intrinsic must be addressed. The FPB, APB, and opponens pollicis can be released through the same incision in the thenar crease. The muscles

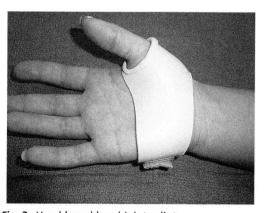

Fig. 3. Hand-based basal joint splint.

are released from their origins on the transverse carpal ligament and the thumb is extended to allow radial migration of the muscles. The first dorsal interosseous may also be released from either its insertion or origin. However, release from its first metacarpal origin is preferred to avoid intrinsic dysfunction of the index finger.[27,47,48] The release can be performed through the index web or, as Matev[42] describes, through the thenar incision for the adductor release.

In patients with uncontrolled spasticity, an ulnar motor nerve neurectomy performed at Guyon's canal may be performed instead of or in addition to the muscle releases.

Skin

The method of skin coverage following contracture release must be considered preoperatively to ensure availability of donor sites and possible need for distant surgery. The preoperative determination between spasticity and contracture takes on great importance here because spasticity alone may not involve any skin tightness. For minor contractures z-plasties can be effective in increasing the thumb-index finger span and restoring an adequate first web space. There is a variety of z-plasty techniques available, with the decision of which to use based on the amount of length increase needed and comfort of the surgeon. Increasing the angle of the z-plasty increases length gained but also increases difficulty of skin closure, and thus for a 2-limb z-plasty the authors prefer a 60° angle. Mustarde[49] originally described the "jumping man flap" modified by Hirshowitz into a 5-limb flap combining a double z-plasty and Y-V advancement.[50] The 4-limb z-plasty is commonly used and preferred when more length and deepening are needed, and has been found to double the deepening when compared with the 5-flap z-plasty.[51]

If inadequate skin is available, alternative reconstructive options are required and should be determined preoperatively. Such options may include skin grafting, local flaps, or distant flaps. When skin grafting is used, defects should be created before harvesting because of the difficulty in estimating skin requirements. If a tourniquet is used it should be let down to assess viability of the wound bed. In general, full-thickness skin grafting is preferable in the web spaces, as they contract less than split-thickness grafts.[52] Care should be taken to select donor sites with similar color and texture to the recipient site. The ulnar eminence is readily available in the same operative field and provides a similar type of skin, but limited in quantity. The medial upper arm and groin are

useful for larger defects, but care should be taken when using the groin region in children in order to avoid areas that may later grow pubic hair.[53]

Rotational flaps from the thumb, index finger, and dorsum of the wrist have been well described. Spinner[54] described a commonly used flap using skin from the dorsum of the index finger rotated into the web-space defect. Skin from the dorsum of the thumb can be used similarly.[55] Donor defects are closed primarily or with use of split-thickness or full-thickness skin grafts.

When more significant coverage is required the radial artery forearm flap, posterior interosseous artery flap, groin flap, and cross-arm flap may be considered. The radial artery forearm flap has the advantage of being in the operative field and can be harvested with fascia alone, thus with no donor defect or with a skin pedicle that may require grafting. The groin flap offers large amounts of tissue with minimal donor defect, but requires that the hand be affixed to the groin region for up to 3 weeks, which is problematic in children.

A wide variety of free flaps has been used, including the dorsalis pedis, temporalis, lateral arm, and parascapular free flaps.[53] Of these the lateral arm flap is the authors' preferred technique, as it is easily harvested, may often be closed primarily, and offers an appropriate soft-tissue bulk (**Fig. 5**).

Trapeziometacarpal Capsulectomy and Trapezial Excision

If after intrinsic releases capsular contraction limits basal joint motion, selective releases of the basal joint ligaments may be needed; these include the deep anterior oblique, dorsal radial capsular, and ulnar ligaments. Pinning of the basal joint in a more functional position following release may be needed if stability is not maintained. In certain cases where release does not allow correction of

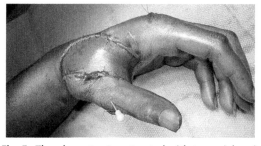

Fig. 5. Thumb contracture treated with trapezial excision and a lateral arm free flap for web-space reconstruction.

the contracture, such as results from severe burn injuries, trapezial excision will provide increased mobility and positioning of the thumb.

With first CMC arthritis or rheumatoid arthritis associated with thumb adduction contractures, excision of the trapezium often corrects contractures. Unlike other causes of thumb contracture, in these cases the skin remains uninvolved and need not be addressed surgically. If following excision of the trapezium web-space distance is not corrected, further release of soft tissues is warranted. In patients with rheumatoid arthritis and thumb adduction contractures, Kessler[56] noted that the adductor pollicis was not contracted but rather the adductor aponeurosis was found to be contracted over the muscle bellies as a tight fibrous band, and advocated release of the adductor aponeurosis as part of the thumb reconstruction.

Neurectomy

Neurectomy of the deep branch of the ulnar nerve distal to Guyon's canal has been described in patients with flexion contractures of the digits as an adjunct to releases and transfers to prevent intrinsic contracture plus deformities in the hand.[57] Neurectomy results in complete loss of intrinsic function, and should therefore only be used when thumb and finger function are not anticipated but rather are used for hygiene purposes. The procedure is performed by making an incision over Guyon's canal then identifying the neurovascular bundle. A nerve stimulator can be helpful to confirm localization of the deep motor branch as it travels around the hook of the hamate. A segment of nerve is excised, taking care not to injure the sensory branch or the ulnar artery.

To prevent intrinsic contractures of the thumb in patients with spastic upper motor neuron syndromes, Pappas and colleagues[58] added a neurectomy of the recurrent motor branch of the median nerve in patients undergoing wrist arthrodesis and superficialis to profundus tendon transfers to address intrinsic spastic thumb-in-palm deformities caused by spastic thenar muscles. The group of patients with median motor nerve neurectomies developed decreased incidence of thumb-in-palm deformities, obviating the need for thumb intrinsic release procedures in this select group of patients with nonfunctional hands.

Tendon Transfers

Tendon transfers cannot be used to correct a fixed contracture, and this is in fact a contraindication for its use. In circumstances where a thumb condition leads to both contracture and weakness, such as in CP or congenital clasped thumb, a combination of contracture release and tendon transfer may be used to correct both symptoms. Tendon transfers are customized to patient needs and must adhere to general principles of tendon transfers in other areas, including availability and expendability of donor muscles, appropriate excursion and strength, and synergy of transferred tendons.

Arthrodesis

Early described procedures for thumb-in-palm deformities used intermetacarpal bone blocks to stabilize the thumb, sacrificing thumb movement and function.[27] CMC arthrodesis in cases where stability is needed maintains function by allowing some movement at the scaphotrapezial joint.[27] CMC fusions have mostly been described for younger patients with osteoarthritis or posttraumatic arthritis of the basal joint. Bamberger and colleagues[59] performed the procedure in 37 patients and had satisfactory results even in older patients. Other than for arthritic conditions, CMC arthrodesis is indicated when stability is needed following soft-tissue releases for severe trauma and burn injuries.

Stability at the MP joint must be present following any thumb procedure to allow proper function. In CMC osteoarthritis or rheumatoid arthritis, adduction contractures can lead to compensatory MP hyperextension (**Fig. 6**). Instability of the MP joint or hyperextension greater than 20° is an indication for fusion or volar plate advancement. When transferring tendons to augment weak extensors in CP patients, hyperextension deformities of the MP greater than 20° require joint stabilization to avoid

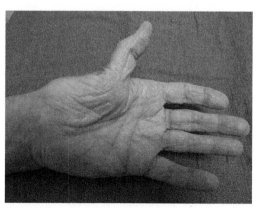

Fig. 6. Clinical appearance of a patient with basal joint arthritis and a thumb adduction contracture leading to a compensatory hyperextension of the thumb metacarpophalangeal (MP) joint.

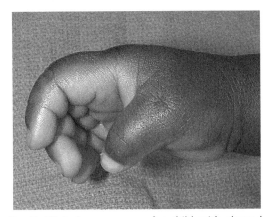

Fig. 7. Clinical appearance of a child with clasped-thumb deformity.

further MP hyperextension and compensatory metacarpal adduction.[27,60]

CASE ILLUSTRATION

A 3-year-old child with congenital clasped thumb deformity presented with an adduction contracture of the metacarpal, MP flexion deformity, absence of thumb extensors, and a web-space contracture (**Fig. 7**). A one-stage surgical procedure was performed to address all conditions including a 4-limb z-plasty, intrinsic releases, and a flexor digitorum superficialis to EPL tendon transfer (**Fig. 8**).

SUMMARY

A wide range of conditions can lead to intrinsic contractures of the thumb. A thorough understanding of the normal and pathologic anatomy as well as the disease processes and their effect

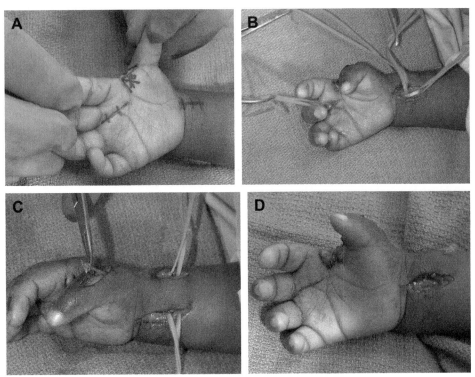

Fig. 8. (*A*) Incisions marked before incision, including 4-limb z-plasty to address web-space contracture and perform intrinsic release, incision over the middle finger MP joint to harvest the flexor digitorum superficialis (FDS), incision in the distal forearm to reroute the FDS to a thumb extensor, Incision over first dorsal compartment (not seen) to route FDS around first dorsal compartment tendons to act as pulley, and incision over dorsum of thumb MP (not seen) to perform transfer into the extensor mechanism. (*B*) FDS to the middle finger located in both wounds in preparation for harvesting. Web-space incision completed along with intrinsic releases of tight muscles. (*C*) FDS rerouted subcutaneously across the radial side of the forearm using the abductor pollicis longus and extensor pollicis brevis tendons as pulleys then brought subcutaneously to the dorsum of the thumb for transfer into the extensor mechanism. (*D*) Final position of the thumb showing correction of clasped-thumb deformity and web-space contracture.

on thumb function is essential in understanding and treating these contractures. Because intrinsic contractures of the thumb rarely present in isolation, a patient-specific approach based on functional needs is required. Prevention of iatrogenic contractures and progression of predictable contractures regardless of etiology is the health care provider's primary responsibility.

REFERENCES

1. Ferretti BL, Cadle KJ, Fahnestock L, editors. Stedman's medical dictionary online. Based on Stedman's medical dictionary. 28th edition. Baltimore (MD): Lippincott Williams & Wilkins; 2006. Available at: http://www.stedmansonline.com/content.aspx?id=mlrC1500020054&termtype=t; 2006. Accessed June 28, 2011.

2. Littler JW. The hand and wrist. In: Howarth MB, editor. A textbook of orthopedics. Philadelphia: W.B. Saunders; 1952. p. 244–96.

3. Dellaero DT, Levin LS. Compartment syndrome of the hand. Etiology, diagnosis, and treatment. Am J Orthop (Belle Mead NJ) 1996;25(6):404–8.

4. Bunnell S. Ischaemic contracture, local, in the hand. J Bone Joint Surg Am 1953;35(1):88–101.

5. Tubiana R. Dupuytren's disease of the radial side of the hand. Hand Clin 1999;15(1):149–59.

6. McCarroll HR Jr. Congenital flexion deformities of the thumb. Hand Clin 1985;1(3):567–75.

7. Mih AD. Congenital clasped thumb. Hand Clin 1998; 14(1):77–84.

8. Wilkie AO, Slaney SF, Oldridge M, et al. Apert syndrome results from localized mutations of FGFR2 and is allelic with Crouzon syndrome. Nat Genet 1995;9(2):165–72.

9. Mayou BJ, Kahn U. Epidermolysis bullosa of the hand. In: Gupta A, Kay S, Sheker L, editors. The growing hand. London: Mosby; 2000. p. 425–9.

10. Jain A, Brennan F, Troeberg L, et al. The role of matrix metalloproteinases in rheumatoid tendon disease. J Hand Surg Am 2002;27(6):1059–64.

11. Akhavani MA, Paleolog EM, Kang N. Muscle hypoxia in rheumatoid hands: does it play a role in ulnar drift? J Hand Surg Am 2011;36(4):677–85.

12. Nalebuff EA. Diagnosis, classification and management of rheumatoid thumb deformities. Bull Hosp Joint Dis 1968;29(2):119–37.

13. Dray GJ. The hand in systemic lupus erythematosus. Hand Clin 1989;5(2):145–55.

14. Dray GJ, Millender LH, Nalebuff EA, et al. The surgical treatment of hand deformities in systemic lupus erythematosus. J Hand Surg Am 1981;6(4):339–45.

15. Feldon P, Terrono AL, Nalebuff E, et al. Rheumatoid arthritis and other connective tissue diseases. In: Green DP, Hotchkiss RN, editors. Green's operative hand surgery. 5th edition. Philadelphia: Elsevier; 2005. p. 2049–136.

16. Jones NF, Imbriglia JE, Steen VD, et al. Surgery for scleroderma of the hand. J Hand Surg Am 1987; 12(3):391–400.

17. Jakubietz MG, Jakubietz RG, Gruenert JG. Scleroderma of the hand. J Am Soc Surg Hand 2005;5: 42–7.

18. Day CS, Stern PJ. Fractures of the metacarpals and phalanges. 6th edition. Philadelphia: Elsevier; 2011. p. 239–90.

19. Stark HH, Ashworth CR, Boyes JH. Paint-gun injuries of the hand. J Bone Joint Surg Am 1967;49(4): 637–47.

20. Pinto MR, Turkula-Pinto LD, Cooney WP, et al. High-pressure injection injuries of the hand: review of 25 patients managed by open wound technique. J Hand Surg Am 1993;18(1):125–30.

21. Stevanovic MV, Sharpe F. Acute infections. 6th edition. Philadelphia: Elsevier; 2011. p. 41–84.

22. Patel MR, Malaviya GN. Chronic infections. In: Green DP, Hotchkiss RN, Pedersen WC, editors. Green's operative hand surgery. 6th edition. Philadelphia: Elsevier; 2011. p. 85–139.

23. Sunderland S. Morphologic changes in striated muscle due to denervation. Nerves and nerve injuries. Edinburgh (United Kingdom): Churchill Livingstone; 1978. p. 229–45.

24. Sunderland S. Morphologic changes in striated muscle due to denervation. Degeneration. Fibrosis. Contracture. Nerves and nerve injuries. Edinburgh (United Kingdom): Churchill Livingstone; 1978. p. 246–50.

25. Leclercq C. General assessment of the upper limb. Hand Clin 2003;19(4):557–64.

26. House JH, Gwathmey FW, Fidler MO. A dynamic approach to the thumb-in palm deformity in cerebral palsy. J Bone Joint Surg Am 1981;63(2):216–25.

27. Lawson RD, Tonkin MA. Surgical management of the thumb in cerebral palsy. Hand Clin 2003;19(4): 667–77.

28. Keenan MA, Matzon JL. Upper extremity dysfunction after stroke or brain injury. In: Green DP, Hotchkiss RN, editors. Green's operative hand surgery. 6th edition. Philadelphia: Elsevier; 2011. p. 1173–207.

29. Salter RB. Neuromuscular disorders. Textbook of disorders and injuries of the musculoskeletal system. Baltimore (MD): Williams & Wilkins; 1983. p. 252–84.

30. Cambridge C. Range of motion measurements of the hand. 3rd edition. St Louis (MO): CV Mosby; 1990–1991.

31. Howard LD Jr. Contracture of the thumb web. J Bone Joint Surg Am 1950;32(2):267–73.

32. Caroli A, Zanasi S. First web-space reconstruction by Caroli's technique in congenital hand deformities

with severe thumb ray adduction. Br J Plast Surg 1989;42(6):653–9.

33. Jensen CB, Rayan GM, Davidson R. First web space contracture and hand function. J Hand Surg Am 1993;18(3):516–20.

34. Matev I. Surgical treatment of spastic "thumb-in-palm" deformity. J Bone Joint Surg Br 1963;45:703–8.

35. Davis Sears E, Chung KC. Validity and responsiveness of the Jebsen-Taylor hand function test. J Hand Surg Am 2010;35(1):30–7.

36. Hoffer MM, Perry J, Garcia M, et al. Adduction contracture of the thumb in cerebral palsy. A preoperative electromyographic study. J Bone Joint Surg Am 1983;65(6):755–9.

37. Del Pinal F, Garcia-Bernal FJ, Delgado J. Is posttraumatic first web contracture avoidable? Prophylactic guidelines and treatment-oriented classification. Plast Reconstr Surg 2004;113(6):1855–60.

38. Tajima T. Treatment of post-traumatic contracture of the hand. J Hand Surg Br 1988;13(2):118–29.

39. Wilton J. Casting, splinting, and physical and occupational therapy of hand deformity and dysfunction in cerebral palsy. Hand Clin 2003; 19(4):573–84.

40. Francois Y. Influence of a splint in maintaining the opening of the first web in arthritis of the base of the thumb. Ann Chir Main 1987;6(3):245–54 [in French].

41. Lees VC, Wren C, Elliot D. Internal splints for prevention of first web contracture following severe disruption of the first web space. J Hand Surg Br 1994; 19(5):560–2.

42. Matev IB. Surgical treatment of flexion-adduction contracture of the thumb in cerebral palsy. Acta Orthop Scand 1970;41(4):439–45.

43. Botte MJ, Keenan MA, Gellman H, et al. Surgical management of spastic thumb-in-palm deformity in adults with brain injury. J Hand Surg Am 1989;14 (2 Pt 1):174–82.

44. Tonkin MA, Hatrick NC, Eckersley JR, et al. Surgery for cerebral palsy part 3: classification and operative procedures for thumb deformity. J Hand Surg Br 2001;26(5):465–70.

45. Yu HL, Chase RA, Strauch B. Skin incisions in hand surgery. In: Yu HL, Chase RA, Strauch B, editors. Atlas of hand anatomy and clinical implications. 1st edition. St Louis (MO): Mosby; 2004. p. 87.

46. Witthaut J, Leclercq C. Anatomy of the adductor pollicis muscle. A basis for release procedures for adduction contractures of the thumb. J Hand Surg Br 1998;23(3):380–3.

47. Tonkin M, Freitas A, Koman A, et al. The surgical management of thumb deformity in cerebral palsy. J Hand Surg Eur Vol 2008;33(1):77–80.

48. Tonkin MA. Thumb deformity in the spastic hand: classification and surgical techniques. Tech Hand Up Extrem Surg 2003;7(1):18–25.

49. Mustarde JC. The treatment of ptosis and epicanthal folds. Br J Plast Surg 1959;12:252–8.

50. Hirshowitz B, Karev A, Rousso M. Combined double Z-plasty and Y-V advancement for thumb web contracture. Hand 1975;7(3):291–3.

51. Fraulin FO, Thomson HG. First webspace deepening: comparing the four-flap and five-flap Z-plasty. Which gives the most gain? Plast Reconstr Surg 1999;104(1):120–8.

52. Jang YC, Kwon OK, Lee JW, et al. The optimal management of pediatric steam burn from electric rice-cooker: STSG or FTSG? J Burn Care Rehabil 2001;22(1):15–20.

53. Kalliainen LK, Drake DB, Edgerton MT, et al. Surgical management of the hand in Freeman-Sheldon syndrome. Ann Plast Surg 2003;50(5): 456–62 [discussion: 463–70].

54. Spinner M. Fashioned transpositional flap for soft tissue adduction contracture of the thumb. Plast Reconstr Surg 1969;44(4):345–8.

55. Sandzen SC Jr. Dorsal pedicle flap for resurfacing a moderate thumb-index web contracture release. J Hand Surg Am 1982;7(1):21–4.

56. Kessler I. Aetiology and management of adduction contracture of the thumb in rheumatoid arthritis. Hand 1973;5(2):170–4.

57. Pomerance JF, Keenan MA. Correction of severe spastic flexion contractures in the nonfunctional hand. J Hand Surg Am 1996;21(5):828–33.

58. Pappas N, Baldwin K, Keenan MA. Efficacy of median nerve recurrent branch neurectomy as an adjunct to ulnar motor nerve neurectomy and wrist arthrodesis at the time of superficialis to profundus transfer in prevention of intrinsic spastic thumb-in-palm deformity. J Hand Surg Am 2010;35(8):1310–6.

59. Bamberger HB, Stern PJ, Kiefhaber TR, et al. Trapeziometacarpal joint arthrodesis: a functional evaluation. J Hand Surg Am 1992;17(4):605–11.

60. Zancolli EA, Zancolli ER Jr. Surgical management of the hemiplegic spastic hand in cerebral palsy. Surg Clin North Am 1981;61(2):395–406.

Intrinsic Contractures of the Hand

Nader Paksima, DO, MPH[a],*, Basil R. Besh, MD[b]

KEYWORDS

• Intrinsics • Contracture • Fingers • Hand

Contractures of the intrinsic muscles of the fingers disrupt the delicate and complex balance of intrinsic and extrinsic muscles, which allows the hand to be so versatile and functional. The loss of muscle function primarily affects the interphalangeal (IP) joints but also may affect metacarpophalangeal (MCP) joints. The resulting clinical picture is often termed, *intrinsic contracture* or *intrinsic-plus hand*. Disruption of the balance between intrinsic and extrinsic muscles has many causes and may be secondary to changes within the intrinsic musculature or the tendon unit. This article reviews diagnosis, etiology, and treatment algorithms in the management of intrinsic contractures of the fingers. Thumb and web space contractures are not addressed in this article because they are covered elsewhere in this issue.

DIAGNOSIS

The intrinsic muscles of the hand flex the MCP joints and extend the IP joints.[1] If there is normal muscle tone, a physician can passively extend the MCP joint and simultaneously passively flex the proximal IP (PIP) joint without resistance. The "intrinsic tightness test" was described by Bunnell and colleagues[2] in 1948 (**Figs. 1** and **2**). If the force required to passively flex the PIP joint significantly increases with extension of the MCP or if PIP flexion is reduced when the MCP joint is placed in extension as compared with flexion, the test is considered positive and indicates contracture of the intrinsic muscles or adhesions of the lateral bands. If the force required to flex the IP increases with flexion of the MCP, this indicates contracture of the extrinsic extensor. The intrinsic tightness

test can also be performed to differentiate a tight intrinsic on the ulnar or radial side by deviating the digit. To test the radial intrinsics, the MCP joint would be hyperextended and deviated toward the ulnar side. Lateral band adhesions, such as seen after a proximal phalanx fracture, result in decreased flexion of the IP regardless of the position of the MCP joint. An intrinsic intrinsic tightness test can also be performed by checking to see if passive flexion of the distal IP joint is affected by PIP joint flexion or extension. This indicates tightness or contracture of the oblique retinacular ligament. Lateral band adhesions, intrinsic contractures, extrinsic contractures, and joint contractures may all coexist. In the most extreme cases, the MCP joints are fixed in flexion in abduction or adduction and the fingers have a swan neck deformity (**Fig. 3**). This occurs because of secondary contracture of the MCP volar plate and laxity of the PIP volar plate.

Patients with intrinsic contractures often complain of difficulty gripping, manifesting as "weakness" or "tightness." This is particularly noticeable with objects of large width because this requires extension of the MCP joints (which reproduces the intrinsic tightness test) further limiting IP flexion. Patients are often still able to flex the IP joints due to the flexor tendons ability to overpower the intrinsic.

Causes of Intrinsic Contractures

Traumatic

The most common cause of intrinsic contracture is trauma, which can be further divided into direct trauma to the hand (eg, metacarpal fractures); indirect trauma, which causes edema of the hand

[a] New York University Hospital for Joint Diseases, New York, NY, USA
[b] Washington Hospital, Fremont, CA, USA
* Corresponding author.
E-mail address: npaksima@gmail.com

Hand Clin 28 (2012) 81–86
doi:10.1016/j.hcl.2011.10.001
0749-0712/12/$ – see front matter © 2012 Elsevier Inc. All rights reserved.

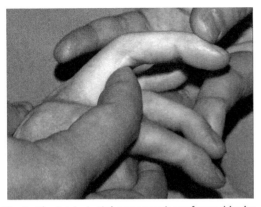

Fig. 1. The intrinsic tightness test is performed by hyperextending the MCP joint and checking the passive tone of PIP flexion.

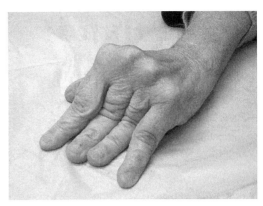

Fig. 3. Swan neck deformity with intrinsic tightness secondary to lupus.

(eg, distal radius fracture, injection injuries, infection, burns, and surgery); and vascular insult to the hand (eg, compartment syndrome). All of these may cause adhesions and/or fibrosis of the muscles as well as the tendons of the intrinsics. The problem is further exacerbated by pain, which discourages patients from performing digital range-of-motion exercises, increasing the likelihood of adhesions and joint contractures.

Mallet finger, either bony or soft tissue, can result in intrinsic tightness because the force of the intrinsics that had been distributed to both the distal IP and PIP joints becomes fully concentrated on the PIP joint.[3–6] This may progress to swan neck deformity and volar plate attrition, further worsening the intrinsic contracture.

Spastic
Another common category of intrinsic contractures is neurologic, specifically upper motor neuron (presynaptic) lesions, which result in the loss of inhibition of the lower motor neuron and subsequent spasticity. Examples include traumatic brain injury, cerebral vascular accidents, cerebral palsy, encephalitis, and Parkinson's syndrome.

Lumbrical plus deformity
In isolated lumbrical contracture, patients experience difficulty with PIP flexion. The lumbrical muscle is unique in that it originates on a flexor tendon and inserts onto the extensor mechanism via the lateral band. Laceration of the flexor digitorum profundus distal to the origin of the lumbrical results in proximal migration of the proximal stump of the tendon. Clinically this is seen after an amputation distal to the insertion of the superficialis,[7] untreated flexor digitorum profundus lacerations in zone 1, Leddy type 1 jersey finger injuries,[8] and flexor tendon reconstruction when the graft has been inserted with inadequate tension. All these situations produce increased tension on the lumbrical muscle and therefore on the lateral band and result in paradoxic extension of the PIP joint with attempted flexion. In such cases, excision of the contracted lumbrical muscle or its tendon is effective.

Other
Arthritis, both inflammatory and mechanical, can result in intrinsic contracture (**Fig. 4**). Proposed mechanisms include inflammation leading to adhesions, muscle spasm, and fibrosis and self-splinting due to painful joints. Patients with rheumatoid arthritis often have intrinsic contractures due to MCP joint dislocations and ulnar deviation.[9]

Less common causes of intrinsic tightness include arthrogryposis and deratomyositis.

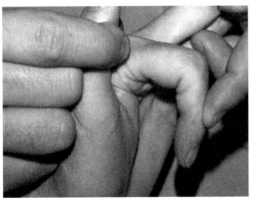

Fig. 2. Checking the tone of passive PIP flexion with the MCP in flexion.

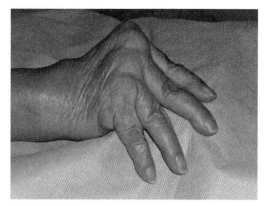

Fig. 4. MCP joint subluxation and intrinsic tightness secondary to rheumatoid arthritis.

Treatment

The treatment of intrinsic contractures of the fingers is based on the etiology.[10]

Initial treatment includes prevention of the problem. In the acutely injured hand, edema prevention is critical. This begins with educating patients about the importance and techniques of elevation. A dependant hand leads to increased edema. In the initial few days this fluid can be reabsorbed; however, persistent edema fluid results in deposition of proteinaceous material, which ultimately becomes adherent scar tissue. Proper splinting and elevation can minimize this effect. Splinting in the intrinsic plus position, with MCP flexion at 70° and IP joints in full extension, is good for the collateral ligaments of the MCP joint but keeps the intrinsics in their shortened position. To prevent intrinsic contracture after distal radius fractures and metacarpal injuries, PIP motion can be started with the splint acting as a dorsal block. For phalangeal injuries, intrinsic stretching and joint mobilization can be performed after fracture consolidation, which usually takes 4 weeks.

Hand therapy is always the first line of treatment in the posttraumatic intrinsic contracture. Edema control massage, elevation, splinting, and compression gloves can all help decrease edema. Hand therapy can be effective for treatment of intrinsic contractures. Therapists should concentrate on joint mobilization and stretching the intrinsics. In mild cases this is done by hyperextending the MCP joints and actively and passively flexing the PIP joints, in other words by performing the intrinsic tightness test.

In more severe case where the MCP flexion contractures are present, hyperextension of the MCP joints is not possible; however, the same basic maneuver is performed.

Hand therapy is also important because it allows patients and therapists to form a rapport that is necessary if therapy fails to relieve the problem and surgery becomes necessary. Patients must understand that surgical intervention is not successful if it is not coupled with an effective hand therapy program. Especially in posttraumatic cases where patients may not have been able to participate in hand therapy immediately after the trauma or because of pain or fracture healing, therapy has been delayed. In these cases, surgery can be seen as a way to reset the clock and give patients a second chance to treat the problem.

PROCEDURES THAT ADDRESS THE PIP JOINT
Technique of Distal Intrinsic Release

Distal intrinsic release (DIR) is the most common method of treating intrinsic tightness or mild intrinsic contractures that primarily involve the PIP joint. In these cases, the patient's major complaint is an inability to make a full fist and weakness of grip. The goal of this procedure is to decrease the intrinsic force on the PIP joint without affecting the intrinsic function at the MCP joint. Because the intrinsics flex the MCP joint, retaining their function is important in patients who wish to improve their grip and make a full fist.

This is accomplished by resecting the intrinsic tendon distal to the transverse fibers that are responsible for MCP flexion (**Fig. 5**).

A 3-cm midaxial incision is made on the radial and/or ulnar aspects of the digit or a single incision over the dorsum of the proximal phalanx. Dorsal sensory branches from the digital nerves branch out at each joint level; these are identified after skin incision and are mobilized and protected. The placement of the incisions is dependent on which intrinsics are found to be tight based on the Bunnell test and deviating the digit to either side (discussed previously). The oblique fibers and the lateral bands are identified and excised. The release begins distally and progresses proximally for approximately 1 cm (**Figs. 6 and 7**). The transverse portion of the intrinsic mechanism that

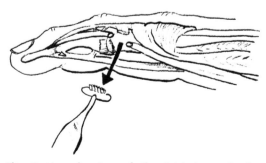

Fig. 5. Line drawing of the intrinsic mechanism demonstrating the location of a DIR.

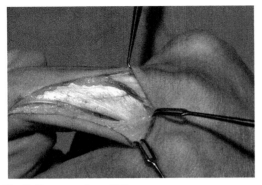

Fig. 6. Exposure for a DIR.

is responsible for MCP flexion is retained as is the central slip. Once the DIR is completed, the intrinsic tightness test is again performed. If the release is inadequate, then progressively more volar and proximal tissue is released until passive PIP joint flexion is achieved.[11]

The decision to perform an ulnar-sided or radial-sided intrinsic release is based on which intrinsic is tighter when deviating the digit and performing the Bunnell intrinsic tightness test. In many cases, the radial intrinsics are tighter and release of the intrinsics on this side relieves the tightness. If release on one side is not effective, then an ulnar-sided midaxial incision is also made. The 2 parallel incisions create a bipedicled flap on the dorsal skin of the finger and are well tolerated without danger of skin necrosis. Although there is a theoretic risk of creating an intrinsic minus hand if both the radial and ulnar intrinsics are released, this is not seen clinically. With the DIR, part of the function of the intrinsic (MCP flexion) is preserved, even if both the radial and ulnar sides are released.

Other causes of PIP extension contractures can also be addressed at this time. An extensor tenolysis can be performed through the same incisions

by sliding an elevator along the proximal phalanx. The dorsal capsule of the PIP joint is essentially the central slip extrinsic extensor and, therefore, should not be incised. Proper collateral ligament releases can be performed by starting on the dorsal origin of the ligaments on the proximal phalanx and continuing palmarly until motion is restored. Intra-articular fibrosis can also be addressed through the same incision and after arthrotomy via collateral ligament release. In cases where scar tissue has gathered in the proximal phalanx neck recess, there is thickening of the volar plate, or there is a metaphyseal spike from a fracture malunion then the area just volar to the proximal phalanx neck can be released and cleared through the arthrotomy at this time.

In cases where the intrinsic tightness has created a swan neck deformity with volar plate laxity, an ulnar DIR can be combined with the use of the radial lateral band as a tenodesis to restrict PIP hyperextension (**Fig. 8**). The radial lateral band is divided proximally and dissected distally. By passing it palmar to Cleland ligament and securing it to the bone or periosteum of the proximal phalanx, the radial lateral band is turned into a static tenodesis that prevents PIP hyperextension by keeping the PIP joint flexed approximately 30°.[10]

The authors have found that using the 2 midaxial incisions can avoid skin closure issues associated with a single dorsal incision and can have excellent exposure of all affected structures.

The skin is sutured and a bulky postoperative dressing is placed. Hand therapy should be started within a week or when soft tissue healing permits and involves active and passive PIP flexion to maintain the gains made in surgery. Adequate pain control, preoperative patient education, an effective therapy team, and motivated patients are essential to a good outcome.

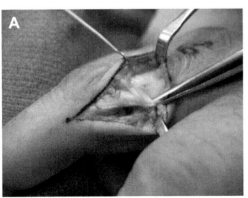
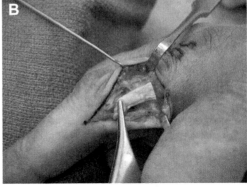

Fig. 7. (*A, B*) Performing the DIR.

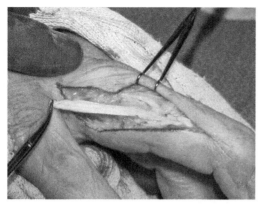

Fig. 8. Distally based slip of lateral band used in swan neck reconstruction to prevent hyperextension of PIP.

PROCEDURES THAT ADDRESS THE MCP JOINT

MCP joint flexion contracture secondary to intrinsic contractures is less frequently seen than PIP extension contractures. When MCP flexion contractures are present, a DIR is not adequate. There are several options for dealing with MCP flexion contractures secondary to intrinsic tightness. These include proximal intrinsic release (PIR) at or proximal to the MCP joint, intrinsic muscle slide, phenol or botulinum toxin type A injections, and neurectomy of the motor branch of the ulnar nerve. The choice of which procedure to perform is based on the cause and severity of the problem.[12]

If the spasticity is secondary to a cerebral vascular accident, some recovery of motor function can be expected in the first 6 months after the injury. In these cases, a phenol nerve block or injection of botulinum toxin type A can help temporarily relieve intrinsic tightness. In cases where the intrinsic tightness has progressed to contracture affecting the MCP joint, then excision of the intrinsic tendon proximal to the MCP joint is the procedure of choice. In cases where there is increased intrinsic tone but good volitional control, a trial of botulinum toxin type A or phenol injection can be used to see the effect of decreasing tone. If the response is positive, an intrinsic slide can be performed. The intrinsic slide is analogous to fractional lengthening of the flexor pronator group. A modest reduction in intrinsic tone can be expected. Because of the few gains and the potential for postoperative bleeding and pain, an intrinsic slide is rarely indicated.

In cases of severe spasticity, the extrinsic flexors can overwhelm the intrinsics, and intrinsic tightness is not revealed until the extrinsic flexors have been released. In these cases, the fingers are held flexed in the palm and the surgery is performed for hygiene purposes. The patients have no volitional control of the flexors. The superficialis to profundus transfer is performed to get the fingers out of extreme flexion.[13] Intraoperatively, once the extrinsic flexors are released, the MCP joint is examined. If the MCP joint can be passively extended, neurectomy of the motor branch of the ulnar nerve can be performed to prevent intrinsic tendon contracture. If the MCP joints cannot be passively extended, tenotomy of the intrinsic muscles proximal to the MCP joint is indicated to allow for MCP extension.

Proximal Intrinsic Release

PIR is indicated in cases where the intrinsic muscles have become fibrotic and no intrinsic muscle function is anticipated. The transverse portion of the intrinsic, that flexes the MCP joint, is addressed in this procedure. This procedure results in a loss of the primary flexors of the MCP joint.

A PIR can be performed via a dorsal incision over the MCP joint that allows access to both sides of the digit. The sagital hood fibers of the extrinsic extensor are identified and preserved while the transverse and oblique fibers of the intrinsic mechanism are released proximal to the MCP joint (**Fig. 9**).

The goal is to completely eliminate the function of the intrinsic mechanism. Because MCP joint flexion contracture deformity places the collateral ligaments on stretch, secondary capsular contractures are rare.

The skin is sutured with nonabsorbable sutures and a splint is applied keeping the MCP joints in extension. Active and passive PIP flexion is allowed immediately. The MCP joints may need to be splinted or pinned in extension (depending on the degree of force needed to maintain MCP extension) for up to 2 weeks. Therapists should

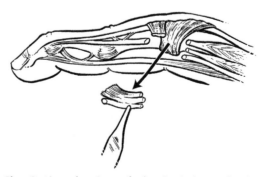

Fig. 9. Line drawing of the intrinsic mechanism showing the location of the PIR.

work with patients to maintain MCP extension via the extrinsic extensor and simultaneously work on improving and maintaining PIP flexion. Developing a secondary extension contracture of the MCP joints is a theoretic possibility but not a clinically encountered issue.

Intrinsic Slide

In cases with spasticity of the interossei without fibrosis of the muscle, an intrinsic slide may be indicated. In spasticity cases, such as seen with upper motor neuron lesions, there is an increase in muscle tone. Hand therapy aimed at stretching these muscles is not effective. A trial injection of botulinum toxin into the interosseous muscles can be used to gauge the effect of diminishing the intrinsic tone.[14] This muscle tone is absent under general anesthesia and, therefore, the intrinsic tightness test is not positive under anesthesia. This procedure is rarely performed because of potential complications, including postoperative bleeding and pain, as well as limited indications and gains.

A transverse dorsal incision or 2 longitudinal incisions are used to expose the interossei. A subperiosteal elevation of the muscles allows the interossei to slide distally while extending the MCP joint, effectively lengthening the muscle tendon unit and decreasing the force of contraction. The procedure may need to be combined with a thumb web space contracture release. Postoperative care involves splinting the hand in an intrinsic minus position for 2 to 3 weeks to allow the muscles to heal in the new position and then starting hand therapy.

Ulnar Neurectomy

Neurectomy of the motor branch of the ulnar nerve can be used to treat spasticity of the intrinsics (discussed previously).[14] The procedure is not effective when there is fixed contracture of the MCP joints but rather in cases where the MCP joints are flexed due to increased tone but can be passively extended. A trial injection of phenol is helpful in determining if this procedure will be effective.[12]

The interosseoi are innervated by the motor branch of the ulnar nerve. Selective neurectomy of the motor branch of the ulnar nerve serves to paralyze those muscles and eliminate intrinsic tone with the exception of the lumbrical contribution to the index and middle fingers.[15]

REFERENCES

1. Smith RJ. Non-ischemic contractures of the intrinsic muscles of the hand. J Bone Joint Surg Am 1971; 53(7):1313–31.
2. Bunnell S, Doherty EW, Curtis RM. Ischemic contracture, local, in the hand. Plast Reconstr Surg 1948;3(4):424–33.
3. Schweitzer TP, Rayan GM. The terminal tendon of the digital extensor mechanism: part I, anatomic study. J Hand Surg 2004;29(5):898–902.
4. Carayon A. Ischemic retraction of the intrinsic muscles of the hand in leprosy (a trial of physiopathologic and therapeutic re-evaluation). Acta Leprol 1988;6(5): 57–65 [in French].
5. Palani N, Selvapandian AJ. A study of management of post-operative complications in intrinsic replacement of hand operations in leprosy through physiotherapeutic method. Lepr India 1976;48(Suppl 4): 748–55.
6. Harris C Jr, Riordan DC. Intrinsic contracture in the hand and its surgical treatment. J bone Joint Surg Am 1954;36:10–20.
7. Peimer CA. Combined reduction osteotomy for triphalangeal thumb. J Hand Surg Am 1985;10(3): 376–81.
8. Leddy JP, Packer JW. Avulsion of the profundus tendon insertion in athletes. J Hand Surg Am 1977; 2(1):66–9.
9. Heywood AW. The pathogenesis of the rheumatoid swan neck deformity. The Hand 1979;11(2):176–83.
10. Peimer C. Intrinsic muscle dysfunction and contractures. In: Peimer C, editor. Surgery of the hand and upper extremity; 1996. p. 1559–81.
11. Espiritu MT, Kuxhaus L, Kaufmann RA, et al. Quantifying the effect of the distal intrinsic release procedure on proximal interphalangeal joint flexion: a cadaveric study. J Hand Surg Am 2005;30(5): 1032–8.
12. Keenan MA. Management of the spastic upper extremity in the neurologically impaired adult. Clin Orthop Relat Res 1988;(233):116–25.
13. Pomerance JF, Keenan MA. Correction of severe spastic flexion contractures in the nonfunctional hand. J Hand Surg Am 1996;21(5):828–33.
14. Tafti MA, Cramer SC, Gupta R. Orthopaedic management of the upper extremity of stroke patients. J Am Acad Orthop Surg 2008;16(8):462–70.
15. Pappas N, Baldwin K, Keenan MA. Efficacy of median nerve recurrent branch neurectomy as an adjunct to ulnar motor nerve neurectomy and wrist arthrodesis at the time of superficialis to profundus transfer in prevention of intrinsic spastic thumb-in-palm deformity. J Hand Surg 2010;35(8):1310–6.

Hand Therapy for Dysfunction of the Intrinsic Muscles

Monica Seu, OTR/L, CHT*, Michele Pasqualetto, OTR/L, CHT

KEYWORDS

- Rehabilitation • Therapy • Intrinsic muscles • Median
- Ulnar nerve palsy

The intrinsic muscles are important structures of the hand and are integral to most aspects of daily living. Loss or decreased function of these muscles can have a devastating impact on people's lives. Often, impaired intrinsic muscles affect the function of other hand structures that are not injured, such as the extensor and flexor tendons. Any disturbance to intrinsic muscles can disrupt the muscle balance and function of some or all structures within the hand, creating a biomechanical disadvantage.[1,2] Damage to these muscles can result from stiffness, muscle imbalances, or nerve injuries. As a result, patients have difficulty with grasping objects of various shapes and sizes, opening doors or containers, manipulating change, placing a hand in a pocket, writing, or typing.

Occupational therapists play an integral part in the rehabilitation of these patients. It is important for therapists and physicians to work together from the beginning to provide the best comprehensive care to their patients. The prescription written by the physician is often the first line of communication between physician and therapist. It should be clear, concise, and include information such as specific diagnosis; date and mechanism of injury; date and type of surgery; precautions; limitations; type of range of motion (ROM) allowed, such as active ROM (AROM), passive ROM (PROM), or active assisted ROM (AAROM); and whether or not strengthening can be performed. Physicians should also be familiar with the different types of splints, such as static, dynamic, and static progressive; their purpose, whether they are for immobilization, protection, function, or to increase ROM; and which joints are to be included (eg, forearm, hand, or finger). With this knowledge, the appropriate splints can be prescribed. If there is a specific positioning of a joint or wearing schedule, it should also be noted on the prescription. With this prescription, the therapists can fabricate the prescribed splint and provide the appropriate care to patients. Physicians should use experienced therapists as a resource and learn from them, ask them any questions regarding types of splints, rehabilitation protocols, or whether they are able to provide a specific treatment such as serial casting. This line of communication works both ways. If therapists have any questions, regarding the prescription, surgery, or whether therapy can be progressed, they should be able to ask the physician freely and expect a timely and informative response. From a therapists' perspective, it is often helpful to understand what physicians' and patients' goals are when providing care, especially surgical procedures, to provide the appropriate care. This information may not be found on the written prescription and therefore an open communication is essential between physicians and therapists.

Occupational therapists play a supportive, but essential, role in the rehabilitation process of regaining functional use of the hand/upper extremity after the physician corrects the problem.

The authors have nothing to disclose.
Outpatient Occupational Therapy Department, Hospital for Joint Diseases, NYU Langone Medical Center, 301 East 17th Street, 4th Floor, New York, NY 10003, USA
* Corresponding author.
E-mail address: monica.seu@nyumc.org

Throughout the rehabilitation phase, therapists educate patients; improve ROM and strength; provide or fabricate splints for protection, function, or exercise; reeducate muscles; and instruct the patient on compensatory strategies or activity modifications. The ultimate goal of all treatment is to maximize function of the affected hand for daily life activities.

STIFFNESS

Stiffness of the intrinsic muscles can result from direct injury to the hand or can occur secondarily because of disuse after trauma. A primary injury to the hand or digits may require a period of immobilization to protect the healing bone, tendon, or ligament. This lack of mobility may lead to joint and intrinsic muscle stiffness.

More specifically, secondary stiffness of the intrinsics may occur after an injury to the shoulder, elbow, and/or wrist. In these cases, patients may be instinctively protecting the injured part by not moving the entire upper extremity, or it may simply be too painful to move. This immobility may lead to a vicious cycle during which patients move uninvolved joints only through a limited, pain-free ROM, eventually resulting in joint and intrinsic muscle stiffness. Decreased ROM and stiffness of the digits can also occur with immobilization by casts or splints, which may partially or fully limit the motion of uninvolved joints and or muscles, and result in joint or muscle stiffness. For example, Colditz[3] suggests that patients with distal radius fractures often use an abnormal movement pattern when attempting to make a fist. Although compensatory and functional, this abnormal movement pattern is the result of both stiffness and disuse.

Regardless of primary or secondary injury to the hand, edema can also cause intrinsic muscle stiffness. Severe edema of the hand often places the hand with the metacarpal phalangeal (MP) joints in an extended posture and the interphalangeal (IP) joints in a flexed posture. This posture has a negative influence on the additional roles of the intrinsic muscles, which are to abduct and adduct the digits as well as to flex the MP joints and extend the IP joints, thereby making it difficult for a person to grasp large objects.

Therapeutic Management of Stiffness

Patients with stiffness benefit from therapy to maximize ROM to provide the best opportunity for regaining functional use of the hand. Numerous investigators have stated that patients who do not have stiff fingers often do better. It is therefore important to send patients with stiffness to therapy to regain as much AROM and PROM as possible

before surgery.[4,5] Therapists use various treatment methods to increase ROM of the fingers, including positioning, ROM, splinting, edema management, and especially patient education.

Patient education

Patient education is important in any aspect of rehabilitation. Patients must understand that therapy requires their active participation. Those who are proactive in their care and perform their home exercise program as instructed do well in their recovery. Therapists, physicians, and patients are all part of a team and must therefore collaborate with one another and understand what the goals are for conservative or surgical management of the hand as well as for therapy.

Positioning

Secondary stiffness to the intrinsic muscles can be prevented or minimized through patient education and with casts and splints that fit properly. It is common to see patients with a distal radius fracture who are in an ill-fitting cast that does not allow mobility of the MP joints or is too tight. Cast placement by physicians that allows full or almost full ROM of all joints of the hand, especially MP flexion and abduction of all digits, enables maximum functional hand use, while still protecting a fracture or ligamentous repair. Use of slings should be limited because patients are often afraid to move their uninvolved joints because of pain or simply not knowing that they are allowed to for fear of reinjury. Use of the sling only encourages immobility and can amplify problems of stiffness and healing. Therefore, patient education is an essential part in the prevention of stiffness and must be provided and reinforced from the beginning. Patients must be instructed and should ideally gain an understanding of the importance of moving the uninvolved joints.

ROM

The goal of occupational therapists working with patients who have secondary stiffness is to regain ROM of the fingers for functional use of the hand. To provide the most effective treatment, therapists must perform a thorough evaluation of the patient that includes determining whether the patient has joint stiffness or intrinsic tightness. There are numerous resources that describe how to distinguish between joint stiffness and intrinsic tightness.[1,6,7]

After a thorough evaluation to determine the possible causes of stiffness or tightness, therapists use a variety of methods to achieve increased ROM. Patients who are immobilized must be instructed to maintain the ROM of the MP joints and elasticity of the intrinsics of all their digits while still casted. They are instructed on methods to achieve or increase AROM of uninvolved joints, including tendon gliding for finger movement (**Fig. 1**).

Treatment to address joint stiffness and intrinsic tightness include both AROM and PROM. Isolated and composite PROM is performed to all joints of the fingers in flexion and extension, as well as finger abduction. If a patient presents with a proximal interphalangeal (PIP) joint flexion contracture, static progressive, dynamic splinting, or serial casting can be used as an adjunct to the therapy program (**Fig. 2**). Dynamic splinting is initially worn for intervals of 10 to 15 minutes throughout the day, with gradual increase of wearing tolerance. For patients who have a greater degree of stiffness at their PIP joint, serial casting can be beneficial. Serial casts of the PIP joint are applied on a weekly basis after maximal extension is achieved through both AROM and PROM during the treatment session. With the cast in place, patients are instructed to actively flex the distal IP (DIP) joint as part of the home program.

Several methods can be used to stretch the intrinsics, depending on the severity of stiffness or tightness. When stretching the intrinsic muscles, the MPs are extended and the PIP and DIP joints are passively flexed into a hook position. Static progressive and dynamic splints can be fabricated to mobilize joints and provide low-load prolonged stretching of the intrinsic muscles (**Fig. 3**). These splints are worn periodically throughout the day. Patients are educated on the purpose of the splints, wearing schedule, and precautions including monitoring for any vascular changes or pressure areas. Flexion gloves can also be used to increase ROM.

Treatment of patients with stiffness of joints or intrinsic muscles should always include AROM of the digits, especially after PROM, to maximize gains in ROM. However, AROM of the digits should be efficient and purposeful. Compensatory motions should be avoided to minimize inefficient pattern of movements. Therapists should facilitate and create opportunities for the patient to achieve maximum ranges of motion. For example, the patient with a distal radius fracture should have the arm supported with slight wrist extension to facilitate an efficient excursion of the extrinsic finger flexors. Patients are also instructed on manual blocking exercises to facilitate extrinsic flexor tendon glides at the restricted area by transferring the muscle force to the stiff joint.[3] If joint stiffness is severe and manual blocking exercises are not effective for efficient tendon gliding, exercise splints can be fabricated for patients to perform their exercises more frequently and consistently (**Fig. 4**).

Edema

Edema must be addressed to enable a patient to achieve better ROM. This treatment includes instructing patients to keep the upper extremity elevated versus in a dependent position. Therapists may use gentle external mobilization, Coban wrapping, edema gloves, and compressive stockinettes for managing edema. Patients with severe edema often have their hands positioned in nonfunctional positions resulting in stiff joints and limited ROM. These patients may benefit from splinting to position the hand in a more functional position, with their MPs flexed and IPs fully extended, provided that their joints are still supple. Patients must be instructed on not overtightening the Velcro straps of the splint because that may impede the flow of excess fluids in the hand. Preventing or minimizing joint stiffness as early in the course of treatment as possible enables therapists and patients to focus on regaining active, functional use of the hand. Active ROM of the digits should also be emphasized with patients with

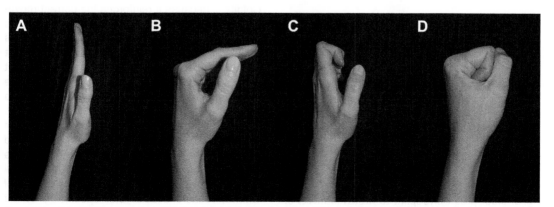

Fig. 1. Tendon gliding exercises. (*A*) Straight fist, (*B*) table top, (*C*) hook fist, (*D*) full composite fist.

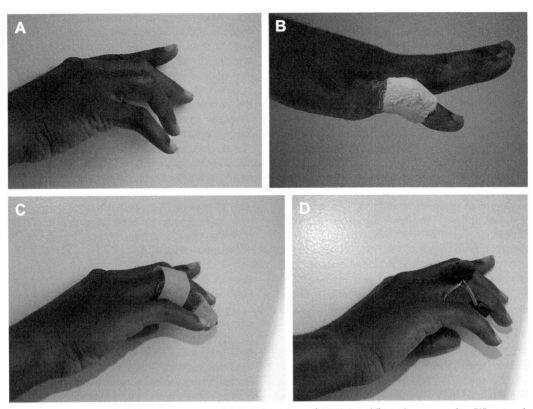

Fig. 2. (A) PIP joint with flexion contracture, (B) Serial casting of PIP joint, (C) static progressive PIP extension splint, (D) dynamic PIP extension splint.

edema to facilitate active contraction of the intrinsics, which assists with pumping excess fluid back into the lymphatic system.[3]

Casting motion to mobilize stiffness

Intrinsic muscle dysfunction and stiffness from trauma, disuse, and immobilization may cause inefficient patterns of movement and limit

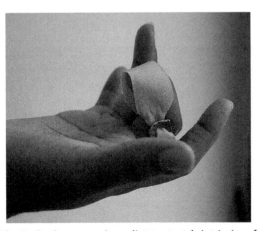

Fig. 3. Static progressive splint to stretch intrinsics of the digits.

functional use the hand. Colditz[3,8] suggests a nontraditional approach to address this issue, as well as joint stiffness, called casting motion to mobilize stiffness (CMMS). The principle of this technique is to cast the affected hand to minimize or prevent any compensatory movements. The patient must then learn to actively and repetitively recruit appropriate muscles to move the stiff fingers, which ultimately rewires the somatosensory cortex to facilitate normal hand movement. Casting instead of splinting was advocated by Colditz[3,8] because it reinforces the correct movements at all times since the patient cannot remove the cast. If the cast is removed too early because of noted improvements, there is a possibility that the patient may revert back to the abnormal movement patterns. It often takes weeks, or longer, for the correct movement pattern to be ingrained into the brain.[3,8]

According to Colditz[1,3,8] there are 4 types of abnormal movement patterns of the hand, and she suggests how to cast the hand to facilitate normal movements.[1] Although this is briefly introduced here, for a detailed understanding of CMMS, readers should refer specifically to her work. In the first abnormal pattern of movement,

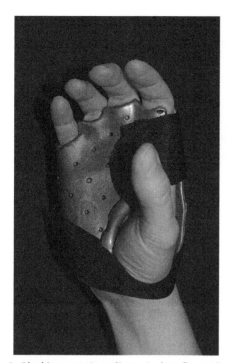

Fig. 4. Blocking exercise splint to isolate flexor digitorum superficialis/flexor digitorum profundus glide to stretch intrinsics. Individual blocking splints can also be fabricated.

mentioned earlier, the MPs flex before the IP joints, because the lumbricals are initiating the movement of grasp. Should the patient show this type of movement, the wrist and MP joints are immobilized in slight flexion in a cast and the dorsal hood is extended to position the IP joints in flexion. This technique is designed to facilitate the gliding of the flexor digitorum profundus (FDP). In the second pattern, the FDP initiates finger flexion first, but is limited because of intrinsic tightness. With CMMS, the MPs are placed in full extension and the patient is encouraged to perform hook exercises to actively elongate the lumbricals. The patient may show the third pattern of abnormal movement where there is capsular tightness or extrinsic extensor restrictions. Flexion is initiated by the extrinsic flexors and the intrinsics cannot provide an effective force for digit flexion because of their suboptimal position. In this case, the patient would be casted to place the wrist in slight extension and the MPs positioned in maximum flexion by a dorsal hood, with the PIP and DIP joints free. The patient is asked to actively move the proximal phalanx away from the dorsal hood. In the fourth abnormal movement pattern, capsular tightness is the main problem impeding the ability to make a fist. The wrist, fingers, and all joints proximal to the stiff joint are immobilized

so the patient can isolate that joint and the movement needed.[3,8]

MUSCLE IMBALANCE
Swan Neck Deformity

Intrinsic muscle tightness, in combination with laxity of the volar plate, as seen in those with rheumatoid arthritis or a previous mallet injury, can contribute to the deforming forces in swan neck deformities. Conservative treatment of swan neck deformities includes positioning of the PIP joints into slight flexion with a figure-8 splint (**Fig. 5**). This position prevents further hyperextension of the joint, while still allowing full flexion of all joints for grasp. The involved digits are also stretched into intrinsic-minus position, in which the MPs are extended and the PIP/DIP joints are passively flexed, to elongate the shortened lumbricals. Strengthening is also beneficial to minimize active swanning at the PIP joint. Therapists instruct patients on 2 intrinsic strengthening exercises: finger adduction and maintaining MP flexion with IP extended, which can be achieved with isometric strengthening and with the use of Theraputty. When performing these exercises, patients must be monitored so that they are not compensating by hyperextending their PIP joints. Should hyperextension be present, the exercise should be modified by performing the exercises with slight PIP flexion.

Literature describes several surgical techniques for correcting swan deck deformities.[9] If an arthrodesis was performed, whether for the PIP or DIP joint, hand therapists can fabricate an immobilization splint. The splint is worn at all times until there is radiographic evidence of fusion. AROM and PROM of the uninvolved joints are encouraged. Initially, the primary goal of rehabilitation for surgical correction that does not involve fusion is to protect the repair by preventing hyperextension of the PIP joint by fitting patients with an external dorsal blocking splint made of thermoplastic material.

After PIP joint flexor tenodesis and lateral band tenodesis procedures, a dorsal blocking splint is fabricated and worn for 3 to 4 weeks. Edema and scar management are performed to facilitate the gliding of tendons for increased AROM and decreased stiffness. AROM and gentle PROM exercises are usually not initiated until 3 weeks after surgery for flexor tenodesis but is encouraged earlier for lateral band tenodesis. Exercises can include, but are not limited to, blocking, tendon gliding, and towel crumbling. Full PIP joint extension is not encouraged until 6 weeks after surgery. When the surgical repair is able to

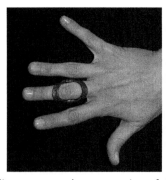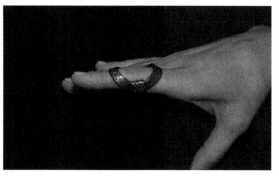

Fig. 5. Splint to prevent hyperextension of the PIP joint to treat swan neck deformities.

withstand increased stress, generally at 8 to 10 weeks, strengthening can begin. Strengthening can begin with gentle squeezes of sponges of varying resistance, isometric gripping of dowels of different sizes, and gradually progressing to increasing resistances.

INTRINSIC MUSCLE CONTRACTURE

Patients can develop intrinsic muscle contracture, whether it be from systemic diseases such as rheumatoid disease or leprosy, direct injury from thermal burns, or ischemia caused by tight-fitting casts, which can result in fibrosis of the small muscles of the hand. This condition results in a detrimental loss of function of the hand. The patient has limited use of the hand to close around small objects with the forearm in a neutral position. They are unable to open the hand to grasp various objects, such as a glass of water, and may be able to pick up objects from a flat surface by using the fingers to slide the object off the table. Patients would be unable to use the limited function of the hand if the intrinsics of the thumb are short, placing it in adduction.

Therapists can attempt to stretch and extend the thumb and MP joints of the fingers through static progressive splints if it is not a severe contracture. Stretching of the PIP and DIP into flexion is performed, as well as abducting the fingers. If the patient has a severe contracture that would not benefit from conservative treatment, numerous surgical techniques are available, as discussed by Harris and Riordan.[10]

It is important for therapists to be aware of the surgical technique performed, whether it be the Fowler, Bunnell, or Littler techniques. Each of these techniques has a different approach to postoperative rehabilitation and complications. Patients who have undergone an intrinsic release via the Fowler method are often placed in an intrinsic-minus position for 2 weeks for the intrinsic muscles to scar down and reattach more distally.

This procedure is traumatic and therapists have to work on scar management to minimize adhesion that may limit ROM.

Some surgeons advocate the Littler technique. During the recovery phase after the Littler release, the hand is placed in a splint or cast after surgery, with the MPs at full extension while still allowing active PIP and DIP flexion. The splint allows functional use of the hand during postsurgical recovery. Care must be taken so that there is no limitation with ROM at the PIP joint. Patients are instructed to perform AA/AROM of all joints of all digits on the first postoperative day in preparation for functional use. Early AROM minimizes the risk of further scar adhesions of the tendon to the proximal phalanx of the finger and encourages functional use of the hand. After the stitches are removed, ROM of the MPs is initiated and any stiffness into extension and flexion is addressed with PROM, AROM, and splinting. Neutral extension of the MP joints is advocated. Hyperextension at the MP joints should be prevented because it may lead to the claw hand deformity, which should be avoided at all costs because the patient would find it difficult to extend the PIP joint for functional grasp and pinch.[10] The MP extension splint should be worn intermittently throughout the day to maintain full extension. When the patient can maintain MP extension and abduct the hand for grasp, the splint can be gradually weaned. Therapists work with patients to increase the ROM to open and close the hand to grasp objects of all sizes and pick up objects from the table, and to improve fine motor skills, such as writing.

NERVE INJURIES
Ulnar Nerve Injury Resulting in Intrinsic Dysfunction

Presentation
An injury to the ulnar nerve can have a devastating impact on a person's ability to use the hand. Patients with ulnar nerve palsy often develop

deformities of the hand caused by muscle imbalances between the intrinsic and extrinsic muscles, often producing a claw hand deformity, which can be debilitating. In a high ulnar nerve lesion, patients may not present with a severe claw deformity as innervation to the FDP is lost, but may develop one as the nerve recovers and reinnervation of the FDP muscle occurs. Another posture typical of ulnar nerve palsy is when the small finger is in an abducted position.

Functionally, patients often have difficulty reaching into their pockets because the abducted small finger gets in the way. In addition, the natural pattern, or sequence, for opening and closing the hand is altered, because the extrinsic flexors act first on the IPs and lastly on the MPs. This pattern often limits a person's ability to use the hand for grasping, because the flexed fingers often push the object away before it can be secured at the palm of the hand. Grasping large objects is impaired because of lost ability to abduct and adduct the digits. Grip strength is also diminished as a result of the inability to activate the lumbricals when grasping, and can lead to decreased coordination when using the hand.[1,2,4,11–13] It is often difficult to manipulate small objects, such as handling change, buttoning buttons, tying shoelaces, writing, and typing.

Another significant functional loss from ulnar nerve damage includes weakness with lateral pinch. According to Hastings,[13] pinch can be reduced by more than 80%, palmar adduction is weakened by 75%, and grip strength is reduced by up to 80%.[1,13] However, patients are able to compensate for loss of the adductor by using the flexor policis longus (FPL). Patients may have difficulty using the hand to open containers and turning a key in the door or car.

Conservative treatment

Occupational therapists often see patients with ulnar nerve lesions who need help to restore functional use of the hand. Treatment commences with an evaluation of the hand that includes AROM and PROM of all the joints. If patients have stiffness of their joints, occupational therapists can assist with regaining motion before surgery. Regardless of the many surgical techniques used to correct clawing of the digits, patients have the best results with good presurgical PROM of their digits.[4,6,14] It is also important to assess the function of the nerve to understand the severity of injury.[15] Any signs of clawing and absence/presence of the ability to abduct and adduct the digits is noted. Patients with long-standing nerve injuries are at risk for developing joint contractures and/or deformities that can compromise soft tissue structures.

Regardless of the severity of the injury to the ulnar nerve, full PROM of all the digits and joints must be maintained to facilitate restoration of the hand as the nerve recovers, or before any corrective surgeries. Treatment strategies to deal with joint stiffness as discussed earlier can be utilized. The rehabilitation of the hand may be prolonged, or may not be as effective, if there is joint stiffness that limits the functional use of the hand.

As with median nerve injuries, injuries to the ulnar nerve also have a sensory impact that will likely affect a person's ability to use their hands. Therapists start the patient on a sensory reeducation program. Details of the sensory reeducation program are beyond the scope of this article.

If the patient presents with a simple clawing of the ring and small fingers, a lumbrical splint positioning the MP joint in slight flexion, to allow for extension of the IPs, is fabricated. This splint facilitates transmission of force into the dorsal hood mechanism of the finger, thereby enabling the opening and closing of the hand for improved grasp. Traditionally, only the ring and small fingers were included in the splint, but some investigators think that all 4 digits should be included. The rationale for this is that the lumbricals of the index and middle fingers are not strong enough to overpower the extrinsic extensors, and over time, clawing of the index and middle finger may develop (**Fig. 6**).[14,16–20]

As the patient shows ulnar nerve recovery, the occupational therapists progress the patient in a strengthening program. In the early stages of motor recovery, the patient actively abducts and adducts the fingers while the hand is on a flat surface. This stage can then be progressed to isometric strengthening by placing an object or finger into the web space while the patient tries to squeeze the fingers together. The function of the intrinsic muscle to flex the MP joints and extend the IPs must also be addressed. One method for isometrically strengthening the intrinsics in this position is to hold a hard, flat object, such as a hardcover book, in a vertical position, while maintaining the IPs in extension. This exercise can be graded by the thickness and weight of the object being held. In the later stages of rehabilitation, as the intrinsic muscles get stronger, AROM against more resistance is added, as tolerated by the muscles. Grip and pinch strengthening should also be included. Theraputty, t-foam sponges, digiflex, power webs, and many other types of equipment can be used to strengthen these muscles. Low resistance and increased repetition is often more effective than fewer repetitions at higher resistances. Slow and controlled quality movements should also be emphasized.

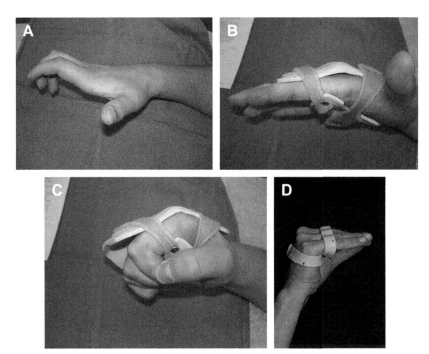

Fig. 6. (A) Patient with ulnar nerve palsy. (B and C) Lumbrical bar to prevent hyperextension of the MP joints in claw hand deformity to allow functional use of hand; (D) variation of the lumbrical bar.

Postoperative management of clawing

Despite the numerous surgical procedures available,[9,14,21] physicians often have a common goal for treatment of ulnar nerve palsy, which is to help patients regain some function to their hands. Some surgical techniques try to create an internal splint that limits MP joint hyperextension to better achieve extension of the IP joints. When a patient has difficulties with IP extension with flexed MP joints, tendon transfers may be performed as well. Optimal communication between therapists and surgeons is important to provide the most effective and comprehensive care to their patients. As therapists, it is important to know which surgical procedure was performed to provide the most appropriate treatment.

Which technique is performed depends on the goals of both the patient and the surgeon. Hand therapists can assist patients and physicians to determine whether surgery can make a functional difference to the use of the hand. They work closely with patients both before surgery and after surgery and often develop a more personal rapport with patients. When seen before surgery, therapists are able to get a sense from the patient of what their expectations and goals are from the surgery and whether they are realistic, how they are currently functioning with the impaired hand, whether they are using any compensatory techniques to perform their activities of daily living,

and, perhaps most importantly, whether or not the patient will be compliant with their postoperative rehabilitation. They can collaborate with physicians and patients to determine which surgical technique is best for achieving the patient's goals. Therapists can also fabricate splints to place the hand to simulate the position that surgery will ultimately place. If therapists know which muscle will be used for a tendon transfer, they can work on strengthening the donor muscles to maximize optimal functioning.

If the goal is to try to normalize the movements of the MPs and IPs to correct deformity of the claw hand, but not improve strength, a capsulodesis can be performed. Zancolli[5] described a technique in which the volar plate is tightened.

When treating patients who have undergone tendon transfers, it is important for therapists to be aware of which donor muscles were used as well as the technique used. This knowledge helps to provide an optimal environment for retraining donor muscles and anticipating any issues that may arise during rehabilitation and that may ultimately affect function of the hand. For example, if a finger tendon, such as a flexor digitorum superficialis (FDS) tendon, is used to correct MP hyperextension, therapists will continuously monitor for signs of swan neck deformity.[14] If a finger tendon is used as a donor muscle, it may correct the claw deformity, but may not improve strength. If the goal of the patient and surgeon is to close the hand with increased strength, a wrist tendon is used. In a summary by Schwarz and colleagues[14] of the various surgical techniques for correcting claw deformity, they noted the importance of also knowing which route was used for the transfer of the tendons. When a volar route is used, it is better for prehension and strong finger flexion. If the goal is to increase finger extension, a dorsal approach is used to limit wrist flexion, which maintains tension on the tendons to help with extension of digits.[14,22,23] This information should be communicated to the occupational therapists via the prescription, operative report, or verbally.

Postoperative Treatment of Tendon Transfers

Protocols for therapy, if available, should be used as a guideline for the treatment of patients who have undergone tendon transfers for claw deformities. Various factors can affect a patient's progress, including edema, minimal or excessive scar adhesion, and the patient's compliance with their home exercise program. It is up to the experienced therapist to monitor these factors to determine how a patient is doing and to progress into the next phase of rehabilitation appropriately. As an example, if a patient presents with considerable amounts of scar adhesion that limits gliding of the tendon, the splint may be discharged earlier to encourage increased AROM. In contrast, should a patient have extremely good ROM a few weeks after surgery, the protective splint may be continued for a longer period of time because this patient may not scar well and the surgical repair may be compromised with increased activity.

In general, during the acute postsurgical rehabilitation phase, patients are usually kept immobilized for 3 to 5 weeks, as determined by the surgeon, with their MPs flexed to minimize tension to the transferred tendon and to allow healing of the soft tissues. After this period of immobilization, occupational therapists can fabricate a dorsal blocking splint to maintain the MP joints in flexion to prevent the overstretching of the repair, which could lead to hyperextension of the MP joint. This protective splint is worn for another 2 to 3 weeks and only removed for home exercise and hygiene.

Patients are educated on AROM of their uninvolved joints, edema management, positioning, and purpose of the splints. They are also educated in their limitations and restrictions, such as no forceful gripping, lifting, or carrying, and no composite wrist and finger extension. Wound care, scar management, edema management, and, if allowed by the surgeon, gentle protected

PROM are also initiated during the acute phase to minimize further stiffness. Gentle protected PROM is performed with the wrist, and all joints of the hand, in a flexed position to keep the repair slack. Only the joint being mobilized is extended while the others remain in flexion. This PROM should only be done by a therapist.

Muscle retraining often begins when AROM and AAROM of the involved digits and joints are allowed, usually around 3 to 5 weeks after surgery. With ROM performed any sooner than this, there is an increased risk of rupture.[12] Muscle retraining requires active participation by the patient, as well as frequent repetitions. To retrain the transferred tendon, the patient is asked to actively think about the movement the donor tendon was originally designed to do. Therapists guide the patient with verbal and tactile feedback for the transferred tendon to perform the desired movement. Exercises such as place and hold are beneficial. With frequent repetitions, the new motor pattern will be learned and the patient will be able to use the hand for functional activities, including opening the hand to grasp objects of various shapes and sizes.

Full PROM of joints is ideally obtained before surgery to maximize the likelihood of a better functional outcome for the hand. If there is soft tissue shortening and/or joint contracture, a patient may create too much tension when opening or closing the hand, and therefore risk rupturing the tendon repair. If a patient does not have full passive motion, because of joint stiffness or soft tissue shortening, care must be used when performing PROM so the tendon transfer is not overstretched. PROM is generally not started until around 6 to 8 weeks, when the tendons are able to withstand greater amounts of stress. At this time, patients are encouraged to use their hands for light functional activities, such as bathing or grasping light objects. At 8 to 12 weeks, the strengthening phase can be safely initiated.[5,12] Foam sponges, Theraputty, or a hand helper can be used for increasing the resistance as the muscles get stronger. Fine motor coordination and in-hand manipulation activities are also performed. Full MP extension may be discouraged by the therapist during the rehabilitation period to prevent hyperextension of these joints. If the deformity is uncorrectable, the occupational therapist can work with patients to find compensatory strategies for loss of function.

Early active mobilization following claw hand tendon transfers is advocated by Rath.[24] This protocol is used following middle finger FDS 4-tail pulley insertions technique for correcting the deformity. During the first and second postoperative weeks, the patient is encouraged to actively move the fingers in a specific sequence to open/ close the hand. To make a fist, the patient is asked to flex the MP joints while keeping the IPs straight. The PIP joints are then flexed to make a flat fist. To open the hand, the sequence is then reversed. Extension of the PIP joints occurs first, then the MP joints. Full MP extension is limited to 30° by the therapist. At the third to fourth week, patients are allowed to actively move their hands and are referred to occupational therapy to increase function in daily activities. At this time, the dorsal blocking splint is adjusted to limit MP extension to 30°, and patients are allowed only to pick up/ grasp objects that weight less than 450 g. Once patients are able to perform functional activities of daily living independently, they are discharged from therapy. At 8 weeks after surgery, patients are allowed to resume light activities, and full unrestricted activities at 12 weeks.[24]

Rath's[24] study shows that there can be a significant decrease in the amount of time spent in rehabilitation, and that the patient is able to return to work sooner. ROM of the fingers is also greater than for those who were immobilized, possibly because of fewer scar adhesions. Early mobilization also begins the new motor pattern's integration into the brain sooner, and better facilitates individual movement of the fingers.[24]

As stated previously, patients with ulnar nerve palsy also have difficulty with lateral pinch from loss of the first dorsal interossei and adductor pollicis. This loss affects their functional ability, such as when pinching small objects and turning a key. Tendon transfers to restore lateral pinch is rarely performed, as most patients do not usually complain of a significant deficit because they are compensating with the FPL and extensor pollicis longus. Patients are educated on compensatory strategies to overcome this deficit by stabilizing the index finger against the other digits during lateral pinch and using the FPL to substitute for the loss of thumb adduction.[14]

Median Nerve Injury Resulting in Intrinsic Dysfunction

Presentation
Median nerve palsy results in a significant loss of the ability to palmarly abduct the thumb for oppositional grasp and prehension. The arches of the hand are compromised and the thumb is adducted to the side of the hand, as seen in the hands of an ape. Patients with severe median nerve palsy are unable to use the hand functionally for grasping objects and fine motor activities such as writing, tying shoelaces, manipulating buttons, handling change, or even picking things up. Those who

have had this problem for an extended period are at risk for developing a web space contracture.[7,24]

Conservative treatment
On evaluation, therapists assess both sensory and motor function of the hand, observing for atrophy of the thenar eminence, resting posture of the thumb in the plane of the hand, and assessing median nerve–innervated intrinsic muscles. Shreuders and colleagues[25] describe the importance of testing the strength of the hand muscles and how it provides useful information about diagnosis, assessment, and outcomes for both surgery and therapy. Any compensatory movement should also be noted.

In the early phase, the goals for rehabilitation of patients with median nerve injuries are to (1) maintain full ROM of all digits, (2) prevent joint contractures, and (3) prevent further injury from sensory loss. To achieve these goals, we often use various methods including splinting. As mentioned earlier, it is important that the patient has full ROM for the best possible outcome after conservative or postoperative treatment. AROM and PROM should include flexion and extension of all digits and abduction of the thumb.

Various splints can be fabricated to prevent contractures and/or to facilitate function of the hand. Daytime splinting should hold the thumb in a stable opposed, but less than fully abducted, position (**Fig. 7**). This splint positions the thumb in opposition and allows the patient to use the hand for prehension and grasp. Nighttime splinting places the thumb in abduction and the splint is necessary to prevent web space contracture (**Fig. 8**). These patients have compromised sensation and therefore must be educated on skin care and inspection to prevent skin breakdown.

As the patient shows returning median nerve function, retraining and reeducation are emphasized. Motor function may return before sensory function, making it difficult for the patient to use the hand for normal activity.[26] It is important to position the thumb in slight abduction and opposition so the extrinsic flexor and extensor do not overpower the returning thenar intrinsic muscles (see **Fig. 7**).[26]

As muscles are reinnervated, the therapist and patient work to enhance the recovery of strength and motor control. Recovery of muscle strength following reinnervation is more complete when physiologic muscle integrity is maintained and proprioceptive feedback is provided. Therapists may use neuromuscular electrical stimulation (NMES) and biofeedback to provide visual and auditory feedback of muscle contraction and

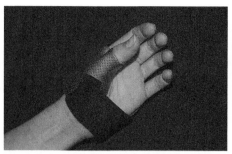 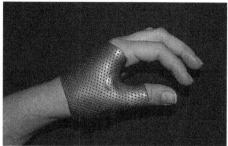

Fig. 7. Opposition splint for median nerve palsy. Velcro strap used to rotate thumb into opposition.

enhance functional activities, strength, and endurance.[27] As the patient shows improved ability to palmarly abduct the thumb, activities to encourage opposition, fine motor skills, and dexterity are initiated. Activities can be as simple as grasping various sizes and shapes of objects or picking up small objects from the table for prehension, or more advanced activities, for example in-hand manipulation of small objects like coins.

Initially, isometric strengthening for tip-to-tip prehension and palmar abduction is performed. Patients are instructed to touch the tip of the thumb to the index finger and apply pressure against each other. For effective strengthening of the intrinsic thenar musculature, the MP and IP of the thumb must be in slight flexion. Patients must be monitored for compensatory movements with extension or hyperextension of the MP joint and increased IP joint flexion. As the muscles become stronger and the quality of movement improves with the patient being able to maintain the position with some resistance, strengthening can be progressed to use of Theraputty and graded resistive clothespins or foam sponges.

When performing isometric strengthening for palmar abduction, patients often have difficulty isolating the abductor pollicis brevis. To facilitate this motion, place the thumb in palmar abduction and ask the patient to hold and maintain position. When they are able to do that, resistance is applied on the radial side of the thumb, just proximal the MP joint. It is helpful to palpate the thenar to see if the appropriate muscle is being used and provide feedback. Patients may compensate with placing the thumb in slight radial abduction. Therapists must monitor for this and provide verbal and tactile cues to maintain the correct position. The patient can be progressed with dynamic strengthening using Theraputty or rubber bands. Rubber bands are cost effective and resistance can be graded by the thickness, quantity, and size used. As with any strengthening, slow and steady with increasing repetitions versus fast movements with fewer repetitions is best for increasing control and endurance of a weak muscle. Exercises should not be too easy or too difficult, but rather challenging for best results. As the function of the thumb improves, therapists often encourage use of the affected hand for functional activities.

As skin receptors are reinnervated, the patient and therapist work to maximize recovery of functional sensibility. Further details of sensory reeducation are beyond the scope of this article.

If there is no evidence of further improvement of hand function over time, reinnervation has peaked and the patient may be left with significant residual deficits. The goals of therapy in this phase focus on compensatory techniques to perform the activities of daily living and educating patients on maintaining maximal ROM of the hand. A tendon transfer may be necessary to restore thumb opposition and functional thumb use if thenar function does not return. On the extremely rare occasion when a physician recommends fusion of the thumb to provide stability to allow for function, therapists may fabricate a splint to position the thumb in palmar abduction for opposition to simulate fusion. This position allows the patient to have an idea of the ramifications of thumb fusion. As mentioned earlier, this is extremely rare because there are greater surgical techniques to restore thumb function.

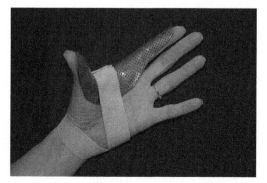

Fig. 8. Web space splint.

Postsurgical Treatment

Restoration of opposition rehabilitation protocol

When the palsy has become chronic and the patient has undergone a tendon transfer procedure to restore abduction and opposition, the patient is referred to therapy for postoperative therapeutic management and restoration of function. Information regarding the surgery, including the tendon used for the transfer and the method, must be conveyed to the therapist for the appropriate care to be provided. Most commonly, the ring finger FDS is transferred to the first metacarpal to restore abduction and opposition.[7,26,28,29]

There are limited specific prerehabilitation and postrehabilitation guidelines for restoration of opposition, and a similar protocol to that used for ulnar paralysis is typically used. Rajan and colleagues[28] proposed a preoperative and postoperative protocol adapted from the protocols of the World Health Organization (WHO) and from ulnar nerve injury protocols. Review of the literature suggests the following guidelines.

During the preoperative phase, isolation and strengthening of the ring finger FDS is performed.[29] A modified resting hand splint can be fabricated to facilitate isolation and strengthening of the ring FDS in opposition to the thumb, because it can be a difficult muscle to isolate when performing dual functions (**Fig. 9**).[28] Green[30] observed that the effectiveness of a tendon transfer is reduced when it is expected to produce 2 dissimilar functions, even when they are not directly opposed.

After surgery, the patient is positioned in a cast with thumb abduction and opposition at the carpometacarpal (CMC) joint and with IP extension for 3 weeks. The WHO suggests placing the thumb sutured to the little finger over a thick palmar gauze roll.[29] Rehabilitation to restore opposition is resumed at 4 weeks for muscle reeducation when the cast is removed and, if not done earlier, a modified resting hand splint is fabricated (see **Fig. 9**). Active thumb palmar abduction and opposition is encouraged within the splint. The patient is encouraged to oppose the thumb to the ring finger with the CMC joint and with the IP in extension. The IP joint of the thumb is splinted into extension to prevent compensation by the FPL, until active IP extension and control can be maintained throughout the motion. Repetitive graded activities progress with different sized objects in a variety of positions.[28,29] Outside of therapy, the patient is placed into a web spacer splint or cast to avoid excessive stress on the transferred muscle. Patients must also be educated on positions to avoid, such as placing the hand flat on a surface,

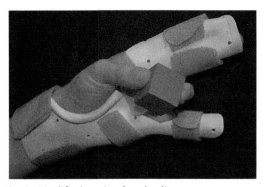

Fig. 9. Modified resting hand splint.

because that can place undue stress on the muscle transfer.

By the fifth or sixth week, the patient is asked to perform prehension functions required for writing, begin unilateral activities of daily living, such as eating and brushing, as well as bimanual hand function such as buttoning.[1,15] Prolonged protection of the hand may be required for up to 3 months when the patient is not exercising. Reeducation after muscle transfers is an important part in the success of any operation. The patient must activate and exercise both the thumb and ring finger PIP flexion for best retraining.

Throughout the postoperative rehabilitation, therapists also work on edema management, scar management, maintaining mobility of all joints of the hand, and progression to the next phase of recovery. Some of the therapeutic activities described earlier in the conservative management for median nerve injuries can be used during the postoperative rehabilitation, when appropriate.

Combined Median and Ulnar Nerve Injury

When both the median and ulnar nerve innervation is disrupted, the patient presents with an intrinsic-minus hand, with possible paralysis or contracture of all intrinsic muscles. This type of injury is debilitating in that the patient is unable to use the hand for any functional activity without any intervention. It is of utmost importance to maintain ROM of all joints of all digits. Treatment of these injuries requires a combination of the guidelines mentioned earlier. In addition, these patients may require a lumbrical bar splint with the thumb included. This splint provides a counterbalance of the extrinsic muscles that positions the thumb in opposition and prevents clawing of the digits. It positions the hand in a functional position to facilitate grasp and prehension, maintain ROM, and prevent contracture (**Fig. 10**).

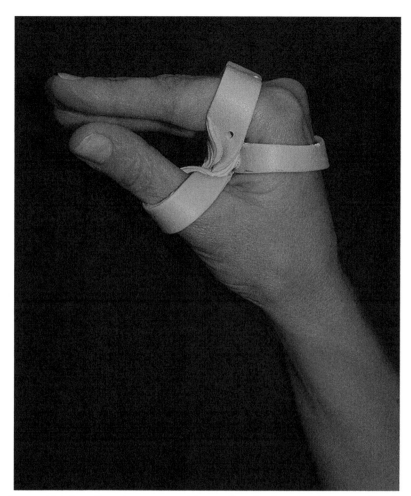

Fig. 10. Splint for combined median-ulnar nerve palsies to allow for functional grasp and prehension.

SUMMARY

The intrinsic muscles of the hand are essential for normal balance, power, and positioning of the digits in all daily activities. Hand therapy rehabilitation of postsurgical and nonsurgical management is vital in the recovery of patients with intrinsic dysfunction. For the best functional outcome, therapists and surgeons must work, communicate, and learn from one another to provide comprehensive and patient-centered care. Patients must be educated on and throughout all aspects of their care, from conservative treatments to preoperative and postoperative treatments. Physicians, therapists, and especially patients must understand the goals of the treatment plan set forth by the physician, whether it be conservative or surgical. Likewise, physicians and therapists must also understand the patient's own personal goals and expectations before any surgical intervention. Therapists interact with patients more frequently and for a longer period of time than physicians, and they get to know and understand patients in a more comprehensive manner. It is common to hear that patients do not understand the purpose of the surgery or have an unrealistic goal of how their hand will function after surgery and rehabilitation. It is important that patients know from the beginning that they are an integral part of a team and it is expected that they will take an active role in their recovery. The success or lack of success in the recovery of the hand depends on their participation in the rehabilitation process and follow-through of instructions provided by therapists and physicians.

REFERENCES

1. Dell P, Sforzo CR. Ulnar intrinsic anatomy and dysfunction. J Hand Ther 2005;18(2):198–207.
2. Brandsma JW, Andersen JG. Primary defects of the hand with intrinsic paralysis [special article]. British Leprosy Relief Association 1984;55:103–6.

3. Colditz JC. Therapist's management of the stiff hand. In: Hunter JM, Mackin EJ, Callahan AD, et al, editors. 5th edition, Rehabilitation of the hand and upper extremity, vol. 1. St Louis (MO): Mosby; 2002. p. 1021–49.

4. Tse R, Hentz VR, Yao J. Late reconstruction for ulnar nerve palsy. Hand Clin 2007;23:373–92.

5. Zancolli EA. Claw-hand caused by paralysis of the intrinsic muscles: a simple surgical procedure for its correction. J Bone Joint Surg Am 1957;39(5): 1076–80.

6. Aulicino PL. Clinical evaluation of the hand. In: Hunter JM, Mackin EJ, Callahan AD, et al, editors. 5th edition, Rehabilitation of the hand and upper extremity, vol. 1. St Louis: Mosby; 2002. p. 120–42.

7. Beasley RW. Surgery of the hand. New York: Thieme; 2003. p. 26–50.

8. Colditz JC. A new technique for casting motion to mobilize stiffness (CMMS) [Course notes]. New York; 2003.

9. Boyer MI, Gelberman RH. Operative correction of swan-neck and boutonniere deformities in the rheumatoid hand. J Am Acad Orthop Surg 1999;7(2): 92–100.

10. Harris C, Riordan D. Intrinsic contracture in the hand and its surgical treatment. J Bone Joint Surg Am 1954;36(1):10–20.

11. Goldfarb CA, Stern PJ. Low ulnar nerve palsy. J Am Soc Surg Hand 2003;3(1):14–26.

12. Bell-Krotoski JA. Preoperative and postoperative management of tendon transfers after median and ulnar nerve injury. In: Hunter JM, Mackin EJ, Callahan AD, et al, editors. 5th edition, Rehabilitation of the hand and upper extremity, vol. 1. St Louis (MO): Mosby; 2002. p. 799–820.

13. Hastings H. Tendon transfers for the upper extremity. In: Programs and Abstracts of Hand Care 2010 Conference. Indianapolis; October 28–30, 2010. p. 157–71.

14. Schwarz RJ, Brandsma JW, Giurintano DJ. A review of the biomechanics of intrinsic replacement in ulnar palsy. J Hand Surg Eur Vol 2010; 35(2):94–102.

15. Goldman SB, Brininger TL, Schrader JW, et al. A review of clinical tests and signs for the assessment of ulnar neuropathy. J Hand Ther 2009;22:209–20.

16. Omer GE. Early tendon transfers in the rehabilitation of median, radial and ulnar palsies. Ann Chir Main 1982;1(2):187–90.

17. Srinivasan H. Movement patterns of interosseous-minus fingers. J Bone Joint Surg Am 1979;61: 557–61.

18. Chan R. Splinting for the peripheral nerve injury in the upper limb. Hand Surg 2002;7:251–9.

19. Shukuki K, Buford WL, Andersen C, et al. Intrinsic muscle contribution to the metacarpal phalangeal joint flexion moment of the middle, ring, and small fingers. J Hand Surg Am 2006;31(7):1111–7.

20. Schreuders TAR, Stam HJ. Strength measurements of the lumbrical muscles. J Hand Ther 1996;9:303–5.

21. Tubiana R, Malek R. Paralysis of the intrinsic muscles of the fingers. Surg Clin North Am 1968; 48(5):1139–48.

22. Sammer DM, Chung KC. Tendon transfers: part II. Transfers for ulnar nerve palsy and median nerve palsy. Plast Reconstr Surg 2009;124(3):212–21.

23. Tubiana R. Treatment of the claw hand. Ann Chir Main 1984;3(2):173–87.

24. Rath S. Immediate postoperative active mobilization versus immobilization following tendon transfer for claw deformity correction in the hand. J Hand Surg Am 2008;33:232–40.

25. Schreuders TAR, Roebroeck M, Van Der Kar TH JM, et al. Strength of the intrinsic muscles of the hand measured with a hand-held dynamometer: reliability in patients with ulnar and median nerve paralysis. J Hand Surg (British and European Volume) 2000; 25B(6):560–5.

26. Colditz JC. Splinting the hand with a peripheral nerve injury. In: Hunter JM, Mackin EJ, Callahan AD, et al, editors. 5th edition, Rehabilitation of the hand and upper extremity, vol. 1. St Louis (MO): Mosby; 2002. p. 622–34.

27. Merrell G. What's new in peripheral nerve repair. In: Programs and Abstracts of Hand Care 2010 Conference. Indianapolis; October 28–30, 2010. p. 79–95.

28. Rajan P, Premkumar R, Partheebarajan S, et al. Opponens plasty rehabilitation protocol. J Hand Ther 2006;19:28–33.

29. Srinivasan H, Palande DD. Surgery for correction of paralytic claw thumb deformities. In: Srinivasan H, Palande DD, editors. Essential surgery in leprosy. 1st edition. Geneva (Switzerland): WHO Publications; 1997. p. 117–32.

30. Green DP. Radial nerve palsy. In: Green DP, Hotchkiss RN, Pederson WC, et al, editors. Green's operative hand surgery. New York: Churchill Livingstone; 1999. p. 497–525.

Index

Note: Page numbers of article titles are in **boldface** type.

A

Abductor digiti minimi, branching patterns of, 23–24
  mechanical action of, 20
Abductor digiti quinti, in opposition tendon transfer, 35–38
Abductor pollicis brevis, 2–4
Abductor pollicis longus, 27
Abductor pollicis longus transfer, for augmentation of first dorsal interosseous muscle, 49
Adductor pollicis muscle, 5–6
  anatomy of, 45
  augmentation of, extensor carpi radialis longus transfer for, 46–47
    extensor indicis proprius transfer for, 48
    flexor digitorum superficialis for, 47–48, 49
    surgical technique for, 47
    to restore pinch, 46–48
André-Thomas sign, 55, 56
Arthrodesis, in intrinsic contractures of thumb, 77

B

Blocking exercise splint, 89, 91
Bouvier's test, 54, 55, 56, 59–60
Brachioradialis, in opposition tendon transfer, 41
Burns, intrinsic contractures of thumb in, 67–68

C

Capsulodesis, in claw hand, 56–57
Carpal tunnel syndrome, lumbrical muscles and, 15–16
Casting motion, in intrinsic muscle stiffness, 90–91
Cerebral palsy, intrinsic contractures of thumb in, 71–72
Clasped thumb deformity, 78
Claw hand, capsulodesis in, 56–57
  clinical evaluation of, 55–56
  correction of, **53–66**
  definition of, 53, 54
  dynamic transfers in, 59–60
  extensor carpi radialis longus or extensor carpi radialis brevis transfer in, 62–63
  extensor digiti quinti transfer in, 63–64
  flexor digitorum superficialis transfers in, 60–64
  Fowler extensor indicis proprius transfer in, 63–64
  Fowler's dynamic tenodesis in, 58–59
  initial findings in, 53, 54
  plamaris longus transfer in, 63
  postoperative management in, 94–95
  Riordan flexor carpi radialis transfer in, 62–63
  Riordan static tenodesis in, 57–58
  Smith sling tenodesis in, 59
  Srinivasan tenodesis in, 58–59
  Stiles-Bunnell transfer in, 60–62
  surgical treatment options in, 56–65
  tenodeses in, 57–59
  wrist motor transfers in, 62
  Zancolli lasso in, 60, 61
Compartment syndrome, 12
Concertina Z deformity of thumb, 46
Contractures, intrinsic, of hand. See *Hand, intrinsic contractures of.*
    of thumb. See *Thumb, intrinsic contractures of.*

D

Dorsal interosseous muscle, first, anatomy of, 45
    augmentation of, abductor pollicis longus transfer for, 49
      extensor indicis proprius transfer for, 49
      to restore pinch, 46–50
Dupuytren disease, intrinsic contractures of thumb in, 69
Dynamic transfers, in claw hand, 59–60

E

Exercise splint, blocking, 89, 91
Exercises, tendon gliding, in intrinsic muscle stiffness, 89
Extensor carpi radialis brevis, in opposition tendon transfer, 41
Extensor carpi radialis brevis transfer, or extensor carpi radialis longus transfer, in claw hand, 62–63
Extensor carpi radialis longus, in opposition tendon transfer, 41
Extensor carpi radialis longus transfer, or extensor carpi radialis brevis transfer, in claw hand, 62–63
Extensor carpi radialis ulnaris, in opposition tendon transfer, 41
Extensor carpi ulnaris, in opposition tendon transfer, 38–39
Extensor digiti quinti proprius, in opposition tendon transfer, 41
Extensor digiti quinti transfer, in claw hand, 63–64
Extensor indicis proprius, in opposition tendon transfer, 34–35
Extensor indicis proprius transfer, for augmentation of first dorsal interosseous muscle, 49

Hand Clin 28 (2012) 101–103
doi:10.1016/S0749-0712(11)00121-1
0749-0712/12/$ – see front matter © 2012 Elsevier Inc. All rights reserved.

hand.theclinics.com

Extensor pollicis longus, in opposition tendon transfer, 41–43

F

Finger(s), and thumb, relationship of, 15
    intrinsic weakness of, problems caused by, 53
    lumbrical-plus, 15–16
Flexor digiti minimi, mechanical action of, 20
    origin of, 20
Flexor digitorum profundus, tendon of, and lumbrical muscle, 15
Flexor digitorum profundus palsy, 65
Flexor digitorum superficialis, in opposition tendon transfer, 30, 31–34
Flexor digitorum superficialis transfers, in claw hand, 60–64
Flexor pollicis brevis muscle, 5, 27, 28
    anatomy of, 45–46
Flexor pollicis longus, 28
    in opposition tendon transfer, 41–43
Fowler extensor indicis proprius transfer, in claw hand, 63–64
Fowler's dynamic tenodesis, in claw hand, 58
Froment sign, 46, 53

H

Hand, dysfunction of intrinsic muscles of, hand therapy in, **87–100**
    intrinsic contractures of, **81–86**
        causes of, 81–82
        diagnosis of, 81–82
        distal intrinsic release in, 83–84
        in lumbrical plus deformity, 82
        in rheumatoid arthritis, 82, 83
        in trauma of hand, 81–82
        intrinsic slide in, 86
        spastic, 82
        treatment of, 83
        ulnar neurectomy in, 86
    intrinsic muscles of, palmar superficial exposure of, 2
    pathoanatomy of, 46
    restoration of pinch in, **45–51**
    tendons, and ligaments of, 10
Hand therapy, in dysfunction of intrinsic muscles, **87–100**
Hypothenar artery, vascular anatomy of, 21–22
Hypothenar eminence, function of, 21
Hypothenar muscles, anatomic variations of, 21
    anatomy and function of, **19–25**
    nerve anatomy and innervation of, 22–24
    origin of, 19–20
Hypothenar soft tissue, ability to withstand force, 21

I

Infection, intrinsic contractures of thumb in, 71
Interosseous muscles, anatomy of, 9–11

as foundation of hand function, **9–12**
    pathologic function of, 11–12
Interphalangeal joint, arthrodesis of, 51
Ischemic injury, intrinsic contractures of thumb in, 68–69

J

Jeanne sign, 46, 53
Joint stabilization, for restoration of pinch, 50–51

L

Lumbrical muscles, anatomy of, 13
    and function of, **13–17**
    relationship to carpal tunnel syndrome, 15–16
    strength of, 15

M

Median nerve injury, and ulnar nerve injury, combined, management of, 98, 99
    intrinsic muscle dysfunction due to, 96–99
Median nerve palsy, opposition splint for, 96, 97
    postsurgical treatment of, 98
    web space splint in, 96, 97
Metacarpophalangeal joint, 27–28
    arthrodesis of, 50–51
    flexion contracture of, management of, 85–86
Muscle imbalance, intrinsic muscle stiffness in, 91
Muscle weakness, intrinsic, and pinch, etiology of, 46
        treatment of, 46–51
Muscle(s), intrinsic, contracture of, 92
        dysfunction of, due to ulnar nerve injury, 93, 94
            median nerve injury due to, 96–99
        of hand, pathoanatomy of, 46
            restoration of pinch in, **45–51**
        stiffness of, 88–91
            casting motion to mobilize, 90–91
            edema and, 89–90
            in muscle imbalance, 91
            tendon gliding exercises in, 89
            therapeutic management of, 88–91
    of thumb, architectural properties of, 5

N

Nerve anatomy, and innervation of hypothenar muscles, 22–24
Neurectomy, in intrinsic contractures of thumb, 77

O

Opponens pollicis, 4–5
Opposition, general principles of, 28–29
    mechanics of, 27–28
    restoration of, **27–44**

tendon transfers for, 31–43
  history of, 30–31
Opposition splint, for median nerve palsy, 96, 97

P

Palmaris longus, in opposition tendon transfer, 39–41
Peripheral nerve injury, intrinsic contractures of
  thumb in, 72
Pinch, first dorsal interosseous muscle augmentation
  to restore, 46–50
  intrinsic muscle weakness and, etiology of, 46
    treatment of, 46–51
  restoration of, in intrinsic muscles of hand, **45–51**
    joint stabilization for, 50–51
Plamaris longus transfer, in claw hand, 63
Proximal interphalangeal joint, distal intrinsic release
  in, 83–84, 85

R

Resting hand splint, in hand injury, 98
Rheumatoid arthritis, intrinsic contractures of hand
  in, 82, 83
Riordan flexor carpi radialis transfer, in claw
  hand, 62–63
Riordan static tenodesis, in claw han8, 57–59

S

Smith sling tenodesis, in claw hand, 59
Spinal cord injury, intrinsic contractures of
  thumb in, 72
Srinivasan tenodesis, in claw hand, 58–59
Stiles-Bunnell transfer, in claw hand, 60–62
Stroke and brain injury, intrinsic contractures of
  thumb in, 72
Swan neck deformity, 91–92

T

Tendon gliding exercises, in intrinsic muscle
  stiffness, 89
Tendon transfer, for opposition, 31–43
  history of, 30–31
  in intrinsic contractures of thumb, 77
  opposition, abductor digiti quinti in, 35–38
    brachioradialis in, 41
    extensor carpi radialis brevis in, 41
    extensor carpi radialis longus in, 41
    extensor carpi ulnaris in, 38–39, 41
    extensor digiti quinti proprius in, 41
    extensor indicis proprius in, 34–35
    extensor pollicis longus in, 41–43
    flexor digitorum superficialis in, 30, 31–34
    flexor pollicis longus in, 41–43
    palmaris longus in, 39–41
  postoperative management in, 95–96
Tenodeses, in claw hand, 57–59
Thenar muscles, anatomy of, and function of, **1–7**

intrinsic, paralysis of, preoperative assessment
  of, 29
  origin and insertions of, 3
  palmar view of, 2, 3
Thumb, adduction contracture of, 77–78
  and fingers, relationship of, 15
  as devoid of lumbrical muscle, 15
  concertina Z deformity of, 46
  functional movements of, 1–2
  intrinsic contractures of, **67–80**
    arthrodesis in, 77
    congenital, 69
    etiology and pathoanatomy of, 67–72
    evaluation of, 72–74
    history taking in, 72
    iatrogenic, 68
    imaging in, 74
    inflammatory, 69–70
    intrinsic releases in, 75–76
    motor blockade in, 74
    neurectomy in, 77
    neurogenic, 71–72
    neurologic studies in, 74
    nonoperative management of, 74–75
    physical examination in, 73–74
    prevention of, 74
    skin coverage and, 76–77
    tendon transfers in, 77
    traumatic, 70–71
    treatment of, 74–78
    videotaping in, 74
  muscle contraction in, 4
  muscles of, architectural properties of, 5
  opposition of. See *Opposition*.
Trapeziometacarpal joint, 27–28

U

Ulnar artery, anatomic variation of, 21–22
  deep branch of, anatomy of, 22–23
Ulnar nerve, deep motor branch of, 6
  injury of, and median nerve injury, combined,
    management of, 98, 99
    intrinsic muscle dysfunction due to, 93, 94
Ulnar nerve compression, 21
Ulnar nerve palsy, 93, 94
Ulnar neurectomy, in intrinsic contractures of
  hand, 86

W

Wartenberg's sign, 54
  correction of, 64–65
Web space splint, in median nerve palsy, 96, 97
Wrist motor transfers, in claw hand, 62

Z

Zancolli lasso, in claw hand, 60, 61

Moving?

Make sure your subscription moves with you!

To notify us of your new address, find your **Clinics Account Number** (located on your mailing label above your name), and contact customer service at:

Email: journalscustomerservice-usa@elsevier.com

800-654-2452 (subscribers in the U.S. & Canada)
314-447-8871 (subscribers outside of the U.S. & Canada)

Fax number: 314-447-8029

Elsevier Health Sciences Division
Subscription Customer Service
3251 Riverport Lane
Maryland Heights, MO 63043

*To ensure uninterrupted delivery of your subscription, please notify us at least 4 weeks in advance of move.

Printed and bound by CPI Group (UK) Ltd, Croydon, CR0 4YY

03/10/2024

01040355-0005